Sports Dentistry

Sports Dentistry

Principles and Practice

Edited by

Peter D. Fine, BDS, PhD, DRGP, RCS (Eng)
Senior Clinical Teaching Fellow
Director of the Sports Dentistry Programme
UCL Eastman Dental Institute
London, UK

Chris Louca, BSc, BDS, PhD, AKC
Professor of Oral Health Education
Director and Head of School
University of Portsmouth Dental Academy
Portsmouth, UK

Albert Leung, BDS, LLM, MA, FGDSRCSI, FFGDP(UK), FHEA
Professor of Dental Education
Head of Department of Continuing Professional Development
Programme Director for the MSc in Restorative Dental Practice
UCL Eastman Dental Institute
London, UK; and
Vice Dean, Faculty of Dentistry
Royal College of Surgeons in Ireland
Dublin, Ireland

WILEY Blackwell

Registered Offices
John Wiley & Sons, Inc., 111 River Street, Hoboken, NJ 07030, USA
John Wiley & Sons Ltd, The Atrium, Southern Gate, Chichester, West Sussex, PO19 8SQ, UK

Editorial Office
9600 Garsington Road, Oxford, OX4 2DQ, UK

For details of our global editorial offices, customer services, and more information about Wiley products visit us at www.wiley.com.

Wiley also publishes its books in a variety of electronic formats and by print-on-demand. Some content that appears in standard print versions of this book may not be available in other formats.

Library of Congress Cataloging-in-Publication Data

Names: Fine, Peter D., 1951– editor. | Louca, Chris, 1963– editor. | Leung, Albert, 1962– editor.
Title: Sports dentistry : principles and practice / edited by Peter D. Fine, Chris Louca, Albert Leung.
Description: Hoboken, NJ : Wiley Blackwell, 2019. | Includes bibliographical references and index. |
Identifiers: LCCN 2018023762 (print) | LCCN 2018024973 (ebook) | ISBN 9781119332572 (Adobe PDF) |
    ISBN 9781119332589 (ePub) | ISBN 9781119332558 (paperback)
Subjects: | MESH: Athletic Injuries–therapy | Stomatognathic System–injuries | Dentistry–methods |
    Stomatognathic Diseases–diagnosis | Stomatognathic Diseases–therapy | Athletes
Classification: LCC RK56 (ebook) | LCC RK56 (print) | NLM WU 158 | DDC 617.6–dc23
LC record available at https://lccn.loc.gov/2018023762

Cover Design: Wiley
Cover Image: © Robert Stone; © Hero Images/Getty Images

Set in 10/12pt Warnock by SPi Global, Pondicherry, India

10 9 8 7 6 5 4 3 2 1

This book is dedicated to all those athletes who have experienced dental trauma, dental disease, or oral health issues that have impacted on their professional, social, or general health throughout their lives. It is also dedicated to the small band of dedicated dental professionls who spend many hours attending postgraduate dental courses on sports dentistry, with the sole belief that they want to support athletes in their pursuit of excellence.

Contents

List of Contributors

Paul Ashley, PhD
Lead of Paediatric Dentistry, UCL Eastman
Dental Institute, London, UK

Peter D. Fine, BDS, PhD, DRGP, RCS (Eng)
Senior Clinical Teaching Fellow, Director
of Sports Dentistry Programme, Deputy
Director of Restorative Dental Practice
Programme looking after the Master's
element, Department of Continuing
Professional Development, UCL Eastman
Dental Institute, London, UK

**Geoffrey St. George, BDS, MSc, DGDP(UK),
FDSRCS(Edin), FDS(Rest Dent)**
Consultant in Restorative Dentistry UCLH,
Honorary Lecturer in Endodontology, UCL
Endodontic Department, Eastman Dental
Hospital, London, UK

John Haughey, BDS
Chief Dental Officer, VHI Dental, GPA
Sports Dentistry Advisor, Dublin, Ireland

Gillian Horgan, BSc, RD, RSEN
Academic Director (Health), SENR
Accredited Sport Nutritionist and Dietitian,
School of Sport, Health and Applied
Science, St Mary's University, London, UK

**Albert Leung, BDS, LLM, MA, FGDSRCSI,
FFGDP(UK), FHEA**
Professor of Dental Education, Head of
Department of Continuing Professional
Development, Programme Director, MSc in
Restorative Dental Practice, UCL Eastman
Dental Institute, London, UK;
Vice Dean, Faculty of Dentistry
Royal College of Surgeons in Ireland
Dublin, Ireland

Chris Louca, BSc, BDS, PhD, AKC
Professor of Oral Health Education
Director and Head of School
University of Portsmouth Dental Academy
Portsmouth, UK

**Lyndon Meehan, BDS, BSc, MJDF(RCS),
MSc Endo**
Dentist with special interest in
sports dentistry, dental trauma and
endodontics, Dentist to Welsh Rugby
Union, Welsh Football Association and
Cardiff City FC, Clinical Lecturer in
Endodontics, Cardiff University Dental
School, Cardiff, UK

**Rebecca Moazzez, BDS, MSc, FDSRCS (Eng),
FDSRCS (Rest), MRD, PhD**
Reader in Oral Clinical Research and
Prosthodontics/Honorary Consultant
in Restorative Dentistry, Director of
Oral Clinical Research Unit, King's
College London Dental Institute,
London, UK

**Ian Needleman, BDS, MSc, PhD, MRDRCS (Eng),
FDSRCS (Eng), FHEA**
Professor of Periodontology and Evidence-
Informed Healthcare
Centre for Oral Health and Performance,
UCL Eastman Dental Institute,
London, UK;
IOC Research Centre for Prevention
of Injury and Protection of
Athlete Health

Robert Stone, BDS, MSc, Con Dent
UCL Eastman Dental Institute,
London, UK

Preface

The study of sports dentistry is a relatively modern specialty within postgraduate dental education that has lead the way in introducing the role of the general dental practitioner in dealing with the specific dental challenges that modern day sports can present us with. Initially seen as dealing with dental trauma, the teaching of sports dentistry has evolved into looking at the role of the dentist within the medical team, how dentists can support medical colleagues at major sporting events, how to introduce preventative measures in the sporting context, the role of oral health with elite athletes, and the importance of screening for common dental diseases.

The changing nature of restorative dentistry is reflected in the demands on dental practitioners to be able to advise and undertake treatment that is appropriate to this particular set of patients that perhaps have more demanding dental issues than our regular patient base. Although the field of sports dentistry is ever changing, the primary objectives of this book remain the same: (1) to inform dental and medical practitioners how to deal with orofacial trauma, both in the field of play and within the surgery environment; (2) to introduce the concept of dental screening, particularly during pre-season assessments; (3) to prevent dental trauma of both an acute and chronic nature, acute being direct trauma to hard and soft tissues, chronic being tooth surface loss as a result of erosion; and (4) to investigate the role nutrition plays in elite and amateur athletes, with a view to reducing the need for them to require reparative restorative dentistry in the long term.

Acknowledgements

We would like to express our sincere thanks to all the authors who have contributed to the contents of this book. Their expertise in putting together this compendium of sports dentistry has been invaluable during the process of delivering what we hope will be a useful reference for dentists involved with sportsmen and women, medical colleagues who look after the general wellbeing of elite and amateur athletes and those allied professionals who witness dental challenges to their athletes.

We would also like to recognize the huge contribution made by Dr Barry Scheer for his foresight in developing the very successful Sports Dentistry Programme at UCL Eastman Dental Institute, London, UK. The programme, which continues to evolve, is believed to have been the first of its kind and has enabled many general dental practitioners from all over the world, with an interest in sport, to develop their skills and knowledge to deal with the specific problems experienced by athletes.

About the Companion Website

Don't forget to visit the companion website for this book:

www.wiley.com/go/fine/sports_dentistry

The companion website features illustrative case studies.

Scan this QR code to visit the companion website:

1

Introduction

Peter D. Fine, Chris Louca, and Albert Leung

This book is designed for both dental and medical professionals who either look after or who would like to be more involved in the care of both elite and recreational athletes. The role of specialist sports medicine practitioners has been well established for many years. The primary role of the sports medicine physician in competitive sport is the comprehensive health management of the elite athlete to facilitate optimal performance – the diagnosis and treatment of injuries and illnesses associated with exercise to improve athlete performance. Sports dentistry is a relatively new concept that is gaining momentum as the importance of good oral health and athletic performance become inextricably linked. For dental colleagues, this book will provide invaluable information about the recommended, evidence-based manner to provide for the dental needs of all athletes. For medical colleagues, the book will give you an insight into dental issues commonly seen with athletes and some guidance on how to deal with certain dental/orofacial emergency situations if a dentist is not immediately present. Throughout the book we shall refer to sportsmen and women of all sports as athletes, and we shall refer to professional sportsmen and women as elite athletes. This book is intended to be used as a manual by the sports medicine fraternity in order to ensure that athletes suffering from dental/orofacial trauma or tooth surface loss as result

of dietary considerations and those who are in need of preventative measures, can all be treated in an appropriate, speedy, and efficient manner. We are grateful for contributions to this book from specialists in dentistry from all over the world. The book is designed to support dental/medical colleagues with the ever-increasing needs of athletes and the increasing role that dentistry/oral health has to play in athletic performance.

In this introduction, we look at the role that sports dentistry plays within sports medicine, the prevalence and incidence of dental trauma in the sporting arena, and outline the chapters that follow. With the exception of teeth that have been avulsed as a result of trauma, we shall consider dental trauma of teeth that are still in the oral cavity, and as such can be considered as cases of head injury. The relevance of head injuries will be considered in the relevant chapter from the point of view of their significance, but will not be dealt with in an exhaustive way as this is beyond the scope of this book. For more information the reader should refer to texts on concussion in sport or neurological information on the subject.

Sports and exercise medicine has been growing and gaining recognition around the world. In Britain it achieved official status in 2005, when the then Chief Medical Officer for England, Sir Liam Donaldson, promised to develop the specialty as a commitment to the

Sports Dentistry: Principles and Practice, First Edition. Edited by Peter D. Fine, Chris Louca and Albert Leung.
© 2019 John Wiley & Sons Ltd. Published 2019 by John Wiley & Sons Ltd.
Companion website: www.wiley.com/go/fine/sports_dentistry

London 2012 Olympic Games. Figures from the London 2012 Olympiad show that 45% of athletes seen in the poly-clinic within the Olympic village or at any of the satellite sporting venues, were treated for musculo-skeletal injuries, whilst 30% were seen regarding dental issues. This high proportion of dental patients seen during the 2012 games indicates the significance of sports dentistry in the current age. Figures collected at recent Olympiads show a steady increase in the number of dental cases seen during the competition period: Atlanta (1996) 906; Sydney (2000) 1200; Athens (2004) 1400; Beijing (2008) 1520; and London (2012) 1800. These figures do need to be seen in context as they represent all dental patients seen during the Olympic Games, which will include a small proportion of trainers, managers, coaches, and ancillary staff. The vast majority are athletes, many of whom use the four-year cycle of the Olympic Games to get their teeth, eyes and hearing checked.

Therefore sports dentistry is not just about treating trauma to the teeth and jaws; the treatment and prevention of oral/facial athletic injuries and related oral diseases and manifestations is a significant part. Sports dentistry has evolved from a recognition that dental trauma is prevalent, particularly in contact sports, at all levels of sport, for all ages, and for both genders.

The Academy of Sports Dentistry was set up in San Antonio, Texas in 1983 as a forum for dentists, physicians, athletic trainers, coaches, dental technicians, and educators interested in exchanging ideas related to sports dentistry and the dental needs of athletes at risk of sporting injuries. Courses, seminars and symposia on sports dentistry are far more common today than in the 1980s. The role of the sports dentist is evolving continuously as new data become available. There is strong anecdotal evidence to suggest that poor oral health can have an impact on athletic performance and therefore the sports dentist has a more educational and preventative role to play than they might have done a few years ago. In Chapter 9 we will look into the implications of athletic performance and oral health. As dental professionals, we now recognise oral signs and symptoms, which can be indicators of systemic disease; recognising potential systemic problems from intra-oral signs is important for all professionals, but when dealing with elite athletes this has a particular poignancy as we are generally dealing with young, generally fit and healthy adults, the detection of eating disorders, which we will cover in Chapter 6, being one example.

For some time the specialty of sports medicine has been well recognised in medical circles and in the sporting world. Professional and amateur sport has been aware of the impact that good medical practice, well-trained medical specialists, and appropriate medical facilities can have on the enactment, well-being, and performance of athletes. The input from sports medicine experts, physiotherapists, nutritionists, and sports psychologists in the care of athletes has been well documented for many years. No self-respecting sports club would be without their professional or voluntary medical support, including the supportive and knowledgeable parents who give their time and expertise every weekend to support their sons and daughters. All major sporting events, like the Olympic Games, football world cups, rugby world cups, motor sports, and equestrian events, are well supported by medical professionals, often with a special interest in each individual sport. There is also a long history of medical professionals representing their country at various sports, including Sir Roger Bannister (athletics), Simon Hoogewerf (athletics), and JPR Williams (rugby).

In the world of modern professional sport, the medical team works closely with conditioning coaches, technical coaches, nutritionists, and psychologists to achieve the best results for the individual athlete and/or team. A lot of amateur sport is similarly well supported, sometimes by enthusiastic medical practitioners volunteering their time and knowledge, but also by well-trained professionals. The first editor's memory of taking a group of 17-year-old rugby players to tour South Africa in the 1990s included persuading the other coaches that we needed a professional physiotherapist with the team to make sure any youngster who really was not fit to take the field would not do so. It ended up that the professional physiotherapist was the busiest person on the trip and she quickly became a vital member of the support team, keeping players fit and more importantly advising the coaches on which players were not fit to play. Most athletes, whether keen amateurs or professionals, will want to continue playing their sport after an injury, therefore the involvement of knowledgeable professionals to support those athletes is paramount. None more so than in the situation of concussion following a trauma to the head. Current protocols about whether players who have suffered a head injury should be allowed to return to the field of play make the presence of a suitably trained person at every sporting event essential. The days of a willing parent saying a player is fit to return to the field of play should be behind us. The importance of head injuries should not be understated and the need to recognise head injuries and remove the player from the field of play is essential for the future well-being of young sports men and women. There is anecdotal evidence of elite athletes having to retire early because of the implications of a further concussion on their general health. There are also well-reported cases of traumatic injuries to the brain being fatal or career threatening. There is well-documented evidence to suggest that an athlete who has suffered a blow to the head resulting in concussion is susceptible to a second episode of concussion, which could be fatal if they are allowed to continue playing. This is especially the case in contact sports such as rugby, boxing, and hockey. Whether repeated concussive or sub-concussive blows to the head cause permanent brain injuries is complex and controversial. Press coverage in the 1970s highlighted the case of Jeff Astle the international footballer, where the coroner ruled that his death was due to 'an industrial disease', suggesting that the repeated heading of a football during his career had resulted in

neurological decline [1]. This case was at odds with another footballer from the same era, Billy MacPhail, who in 1998 lost a legal battle to claim compensation for dementia that he claimed was due to repeatedly heading an old-style leather football [2].

Concussion can be defined as a traumatic injury to the brain due to a violent blow, shaking, or spinning. A brain concussion can cause immediate and usually temporary impairment of brain function such as thinking, vision, equilibrium, and consciousness.

Although anyone can have a concussion, we will focus here purely for the purpose of example on athletes who suffer a concussion. The considerations can be generalized to the general population where there is a traumatic injury to the brain.

The signs of concussion observed by medical staff in athletes with a concussion, according to The American Medical Association (AMA), include the following:

Player might appear dazed, have a vacant facial expression, be confused about assignments; athletes might forget plays, be disorientated to the game situation or score. There can also be inappropriate emotional reaction, players can display clumsiness, be slow to answer questions, lose consciousness and display changes in typical behaviour.

Subjective symptoms reported by athletes with a concussion, according to the AMA, include the following: headache, nausea, balance problems or dizziness, double or fuzzy vision, sensitivity to light or noise, feeling slowed down, feeling "foggy" or "not sharp", reporting changes in sleep pattern, concentration or memory problems, irritability, sadness, and feeling more emotional.

Concussion has been shown to have an accumulative effect in both elite athletes and amateurs [3], and certainly concussion during a game can be exacerbated by an immediate return to play and a further blow to the head. This second blow can prove to be fatal. Some sports, like Rugby Union, have a protocol in place for the gradual return of its players to the game, depending on the

The world rugby recognise and remove message incorporates 6 Rs

Recognise - Learn the signs and symptoms of a concussion so you understand when an athlete might have a suspected concussion.

Remove - If an athlete has a concussion or even a suspected concussion he or she must be removed from play immediately.

Refer - Once removed from play, the player should be referred immediately to a qualified healthcare professional who is trained in evaluating and treating concussions.

Rest - Players must rest from exercise until symptom-free and then start a graduated return to play. World rugby recommends a more conservative return to play for children and adolescents.

Recover - Full recovery from the concussion is required before return to play is authorized. This includes being symptom-free. Rest and specific treatment options are critical for the health of the injured participant.

Return - In order for safe return to play in rugby, the athlete must be symptom-free and cleared in writing by a qualified healthcare professional who is trained in evaluating and treating concussions. The athlete completes the GRTP (Graduated Return to Play) protocol.

Figure 1.1 Current IRB guidelines on dealing with concussion.

Table 1.1 Concussion rates for various sports. Source – 4th International Concussion Conference Presentation – Dr M Turner and subsequent publications.

Sport	Concussion rates per 1000 player hours
Horse racing (amateur)	95
Horse racing (jumps)	25
Horse racing (flat)	17
Boxing (professional)	13
Australian football (professional)	4–20
Rugby union (professional)	7
Ice Hockey (NFL)	1.5???
Following Rugby Union (youth)	1–2
Rugby Union (amateur, adults)	1–1.5
Soccer (FIFA)	0.4
NFL Football (NFL)	0.2???

severity of the concussion. At all times the health of the player should be our prime concern. The International Rugby Board (IRB) have drawn up guidelines for dealing with concussion that are regularly reviewed in the light of new knowledge. Figure 1.1 shows the current guidelines and Table 1.1 shows the concussion rates in several sports.

It is conceivable that a dentist will be the most qualified healthcare professional attending a sporting event, especially at an amateur level, and therefore knowledge about the signs and symptoms of concussion is essential. It is of course prudent to refer any potential head injury to suitably qualified medical colleagues, who can carry out appropriate tests and monitor the recovery of the individual.

Apart from the immediate and mid-term effects of a traumatic brain injury, there is some evidence to suggest that following a blow to the head, there could be long-term implications from repeated episodes of concussion. During the 2015/16 rugby union season in Europe, a study led by Professor Huw Morris featured a premiership club in England who agreed to wear impact sensors to measure the force and direction of impact to the head. Professor Morris said: "The impact sensors have been providing us with data during matches and training but analysing players' blood biomarkers in conjunction with neuro-imaging and psychometric testing will greatly expand this study. This is such a complex subject, we hope this is another step forward as we look to increase our understanding. We have a duty to look after our players, and nothing is more important than their welfare". These 'patches' worn by players during training and competition were developed to address the inconvenience of wearing a wired mouthpiece to measure impact on the head during collisions [4].

There have been attempts to monitor and measure levels of concussion, but without a baseline measurement of individual athletes it is difficult sometimes to detect relatively minor levels of concussion. Pre-season cognitive baseline testing is relatively new to youth sports. It is typically a short computerized test administered prior to the beginning of the season that measures selected brain processes and scores the test for each individual athlete; this establishes the athlete's baseline. If it is suspected that the athlete may have sustained a concussion during the season, s/he can take a re-test. The computer software will compare the baseline score to the re-test score and alert the clinician that there has been a reliable change in the score. Computerized cognitive testing can also be used during management/ treatment, even when a baseline has not been established. The changes/improvements in scores over time help to determine progress toward recovery. It is important to remember that computerized cognitive baseline testing is only a tool to be used by a trained clinician. It cannot diagnose a concussion and should always be used as one component of a concussion assessment.

The Sports Concussion Assessment Tool (SCAT) has been in use since 2005 as a reliable side-line assessment of concussion. The SCAT3 was developed at the 2012 International Summit on Concussion in Zurich; the Child-SCAT3 was released at the same time. The SCAT5 (the latest revision of SCAT3) is a standardised tool for evaluating injured athletes for concussion and can be used in athletes aged 13 years and older. It measures symptoms, orientation, memory, recall, balance, and gait. The SCAT5 can be administered by a licensed healthcare professional on the side lines or in the athletic trainer's office once an athlete has been pulled off the field because a concussion is suspected. The Child-SCAT5 is a standardized tool for evaluating children aged 5 to 12 for concussion and is designed for use by medical professionals. The Child-SCAT5 recommends that "any child suspected of having a concussion should be removed from play, and then seek medical evaluation. The child must NOT return to play or sport on the same day as the suspected concussion. The child is not to return to play or sport until he/she has successfully returned to school/learning, without worsening of symptoms. Medical clearance should be given before return to play".

Balance Error Scoring System (BESS) is included in the SCAT as part of a side-line assessment. The SCAT form (Figure 1.2), includes the Glasgow Coma Score, which was first published in 1974 as a tool to measure the severity of a brain injury [5]. On their scale, Teasdale and Jennet proposed that levels of consciousness ranged from 3-15; 3 indicating a coma and 15 a very mild level of injury.

In the following chapters we shall consider different types of dental trauma, how to deal with trauma both on the 'field of play' and in the emergency room/surgery. We shall look specifically at trauma on young athletes and the implications of damage to teeth in children and teenagers. A further chapter will look at tooth surface loss as a result of erosion and include some aspects of eating disorders, the difficulty of restoring these teeth, and the impact of acid on tooth enamel. Nutrition will be dealt with in a separate chapter, where we will look at the role of nutrition in athletes with an emphasis on their general health and how different sports demand different dietary protocols. We will consider the influences of carbohydrates, proteins, and fats on elite athletes, as well as supplements to a normal balanced diet. As our knowledge about oral health and athletes increases, we shall look at the current data available indicating the importance of good oral health and its potential to influence athletic performance. There is much anecdotal evidence to suggest a strong link between the two; we shall look at evidence to support the connection between good oral health and performance in elite athletes.

SCAT5©

SPORT CONCUSSION ASSESSMENT TOOL – 5TH EDITION
DEVELOPED BY THE CONCUSSION IN SPORT GROUP
FOR USE BY MEDICAL PROFESSIONALS ONLY

supported by

 FIFA®

Patient details

Name: _____

DOB: _____

Address: _____

ID number: _____

Examiner: _____

Date of Injury: _____ Time: _____

WHAT IS THE SCAT5?

The SCAT5 is a standardized tool for evaluating concussions designed for use by physicians and licensed healthcare professionals[1]. The SCAT5 cannot be performed correctly in less than 10 minutes.

If you are not a physician or licensed healthcare professional, please use the Concussion Recognition Tool 5 (CRT5). The SCAT5 is to be used for evaluating athletes aged 13 years and older. For children aged 12 years or younger, please use the Child SCAT5.

Preseason SCAT5 baseline testing can be useful for interpreting post-injury test scores, but is not required for that purpose. Detailed instructions for use of the SCAT5 are provided on page 7. Please read through these instructions carefully before testing the athlete. Brief verbal instructions for each test are given in italics. The only equipment required for the tester is a watch or timer.

This tool may be freely copied in its current form for distribution to individuals, teams, groups and organizations. It should not be altered in any way, re-branded or sold for commercial gain. Any revision, translation or reproduction in a digital form requires specific approval by the Concussion in Sport Group.

Recognise and Remove

A head impact by either a direct blow or indirect transmission of force can be associated with a serious and potentially fatal brain injury. If there are significant concerns, including any of the red flags listed in Box 1, then activation of emergency procedures and urgent transport to the nearest hospital should be arranged.

Key points

- Any athlete with suspected concussion should be REMOVED FROM PLAY, medically assessed and monitored for deterioration. No athlete diagnosed with concussion should be returned to play on the day of injury.

- If an athlete is suspected of having a concussion and medical personnel are not immediately available, the athlete should be referred to a medical facility for urgent assessment.

- Athletes with suspected concussion should not drink alcohol, use recreational drugs and should not drive a motor vehicle until cleared to do so by a medical professional.

- Concussion signs and symptoms evolve over time and it is important to consider repeat evaluation in the assessment of concussion.

- The diagnosis of a concussion is a clinical judgment, made by a medical professional. The SCAT5 should NOT be used by itself to make, or exclude, the diagnosis of concussion. An athlete may have a concussion even if their SCAT5 is "normal".

Remember:

- The basic principles of first aid (danger, response, airway, breathing, circulation) should be followed.

- Do not attempt to move the athlete (other than that required for airway management) unless trained to do so.

- Assessment for a spinal cord injury is a critical part of the initial on-field assessment.

- Do not remove a helmet or any other equipment unless trained to do so safely.

© Concussion in Sport Group 2017
Echemendia RJ, *et al. Br J Sports Med* 2017;**51**:851–858. doi:10.1136/bjsports-2017-097506SCAT5   851

Figure 1.2 SCAT form to record levels of concussion.

The screening of athletes, particularly professional athletes, is a relatively new phenomenon. We shall investigate how to set up a screening programme, which could be applied to professional and amateur sport and which can involve the local General Dental Practitioner (GDP) attending their sports club to advise and if appropriate treat athletes. As with all screening, the idea of screening athletes is the early detection of disease and by so doing prevent pain, loss of training and game time, and to take a more preventative approach to dental diseases. The role of the dentist within the sports medicine team will be discussed. As we shall discuss later in this chapter, there is a higher incidence of trauma due to sports injuries than in other sections of the population, particularly in contact sports, therefore treatment is sometimes required for traumatic dental injuries as well as for a relatively high level of dental caries in the athlete who perhaps has not seen a dentist on a regular basis. Therefore we have included a chapter, which will be largely appropriate for dental practitioners, about building/restoring fractured teeth both directly and indirectly. This will include the use of modern restorative techniques, using appropriate materials, and being conservative when it comes to tooth preparation.

Major dental trauma may involve the pulp (nerve and blood supply to the teeth), so we have asked one of our specialists to include a section on dealing with these issues (endodontic problems). Chapter 5 will consider how to deal with pulpal problems, from pitch-side emergency treatment to the final restoration in the dental surgery. It is important for sports medicine colleagues to be familiar with these issues, so we have included a section about recognising pulpal issues from a non-dental perspective. Of course we should consider closely the opportunities to prevent dental trauma and so we have a chapter on prevention of trauma as well as prevention of tooth surface loss as a result of acid, either in the form of food and drink or from gastric reflux.

Finally, we will look at the requirements for setting up suitable dental facilities at sporting events. These will range from the local sports club perhaps needing mouth guards to be made for its athletes and a phone number to contact in the case of a traumatic dental injury of a player, through to the provision of dental treatment at a major sporting event like an Olympic Games. The latter will involve recruiting suitable personnel, designing adequate facilities, and estimating the likely workload that will occur prior to and during the period of competition.

1.1 The Prevalence/Incidence of Dental Trauma During Sport

There have been many studies carried out during the last 30–40 years indicating the prevalence of dental trauma in the sporting arena [6–9]. To put dental trauma related to sports in perspective, a study by Huang et al., indicated that sport and leisure were responsible for 30.8% of all dental trauma [10]. What we think is important is that we recognise trauma to the teeth and mouth, and the fact that trauma suffered in the orofacial area should be considered a head injury and appropriate precautions should be taken to deal with that. The history of sports dentistry is littered with anecdotal evidence of players having a tooth avulsed (knocked out completely) and the coach sending the player back onto the field of play before anything could be done to repair the damage. In fact an avulsion is quite a rare occurrence [11], but when it does happen it requires quick and effective treatment by whomever is available and appropriately trained to deal with the dental emergency. The importance of adequately accessing head injuries in sport has been a major concern in recent years and should be something that dentists attending a sporting event in a professional capacity, watching their children play sport, or perhaps where they are the only medically qualified person in attendance need to be proficient at. The current guidelines laid down by the Rugby Football Union in England are essential for all levels of sport (See Figure 1.1).

A study by Hendrick et al. highlighted the prevalence of orofacial injuries in female hockey players [9]. Of the respondents, 68% reported having received a facial injury, 11% had fractured facial bones, 19% had dental trauma, 10% reported loosened teeth, 5%

avulsed at least one tooth and 3% had fractured a tooth. In Ice Hockey, Hayrinen-Immonen reported that 29% of all injuries sustained during a match were dental [12]. Ice Hockey is a particularly violent sport where professional players see the loss of front teeth following a trauma as a badge of honour. Obviously the sports that are most likely to result in trauma to the orofacial region are contact sports. In rugby at the non-elite level, Blignaut et al. showed that 30.5% of all injuries were dental [7]; Muller-Bola et al. indicated that 29.6% of injuries in their sample were to the lower half of the face [13]. We will consider the work of Blignaut more fully in Chapter 7 when we look at various methods of prevention of dental injuries. A study looking at the aetiology of paediatric trauma reported that between 1.2 and 30% of all facial traumas were due to sporting trauma [8].

Since the recent success of British cyclists at Olympic and world events, there has been a boom in the number of recreational cyclists. Equally we see a larger proportion of facial injuries with cyclists and 3384 cases of hard dental tissues and 2061 cases of soft tissue injuries were reviewed by Haug et al. [8]. Table 1.2 shows the results for hard tissue injuries and Table 1.3, soft tissue injuries.

Amongst 2061 soft tissue injuries in 1697 patients, 51.9% were lacerations, 22.6% were abrasions, 13.8% were contusions, and 11.7% were hematomas (See Table 1.3).

Table 1.2 Showing the number and percentage of dental traumas due to cycling.

	Number	%
Crown fractures	975	28.8
Root fractures	45	1.3
Luxation injuries	1904	56.3
Losses of teeth	244	7.2
Contusions	68	2.0
Intrusions	148	4.4
Total	3384	100

Table 1.3 Soft tissue injuries

Soft Tissue Injury	n	%
Lacerations	1069	51.9
Excoriations	466	22.6
Contusions	285	13.8
Hematomas	241	11.7
Total	2061	100

Soccer is played across the world and is particularly common throughout schools in many countries around the world. In Norway it was found that from a total of 7319 soccer players between 1979 and 1983, 17.4 % received dental trauma [14]. Studies comparing indoor [15] with outdoor [16] soccer injury rates indicate that indoor soccer players were six times more likely to encounter injuries than outdoor soccer players with similar hours of playing time. Higher injury rates in indoor soccer may be attributable to many factors, including the playing surface, and collisions between players and the walls bordering the field of play. Differences between artificial turf and natural grass playing surfaces account for variable injury rates among adult soccer players playing outdoors [17].

Flanders and Bhat reported that male and female soccer players were more likely to sustain an orofacial injury than football players [18]. This is probably due to the mandatory need for face shields and helmets to be worn in football. (It is worth emphasising here the difference in terminology: in the USA, football refers to american football and soccer refers to what Europeans call football.) They also reported a higher incidence of sporting trauma in basketball, lacrosse, and handball.

Whenever a major sporting event is held it is seen by elite athletes as an opportunity to have a dental examination. Studies undertaken at the London 2012 Olympic Games reported that 9% of elite athletes attending the games had never seen a dentist and 46.5% had not seen a dentist for over a year [19]. We will consider this aspect further in Chapter 8.

The London 2012 Olympic Games also proved to be an interesting opportunity to study elite athletes' oral health and previous history (we will deal with this in Chapter 9).

Whenever a major sporting event is held it is seen as an opportunity for sports medicine specialists to learn more about injuries and how to deal with them. Similarly recent sporting events have proved to be ideal to investigate the prevalence of dental trauma. One such study was conducted during the Pan American Games [20]. This proved to be a good opportunity to compare different sports at the same time; what was surprising was that 49.6% of athletes reported a history of dental trauma and 63.3% of injuries were during sports of which the most prevalent were: wrestling 83.3%, boxing 73.7%, basketball 70.6%, and karate 60%.

1.2   Dealing with Trauma to Teeth

In Chapter 4, we will consider how to repair fractured teeth using conventional dental restorative techniques, but we shall be particularly conscious of the need to be conservative in our approaches. We have not looked at the replacement of teeth that are either lost or damaged beyond repair as the prosthodontic replacement of missing/damaged teeth is beyond the scope of this book. As sports dentists we are occasionally faced with a situation where we have to replace a missing tooth. Several options are available to us, including the use of resin-retained bridges, conventional fixed-bridge work, removable prosthodontic work, and implants. The dentist needs to consider the type of restoration needed by the athlete and take into account the likelihood of further trauma, aesthetics, the oral health status of the athlete, and their willingness to undergo restorative dental treatment. Treatment might be divided into immediate, interim, and definitive phases, which might include the use of any combination of the above

treatment options. In the case of an elite athlete taking part in a contact sport, the definitive treatment of placing an implant may have to be delayed until the individual has ceased playing and an interim measure of a resin-retained bridge be used for aesthetic, phonetic, and functional reasons.

The use of various restorative measures will need to be considered in conjunction with a well-constructed mouth guard. This will be considered in Chapter 7.

1.3   The Role of Saliva in Tooth Surface Loss

We have not included a separate chapter in the book on saliva, but we do consider the role of hydration with athletes in some detail in Chapters 7 and 8. It is worth mentioning that saliva has a major role to play in hydration, and so the testing of a patient's saliva is important, particularly when planning restorative treatment and instigating preventative measures. The important aspects to consider are: the buffering capacity of saliva, saliva flow rates, level of hydration as indicated by saliva volume, the consistency of saliva as this can be an issue if saliva is too viscous and does not naturally wash the dentition, the quantity of saliva being reduced due to medication, i.e. systemic bronchodilators, cardiac anti-arrhythmics, expectorants, and tranquillisers. There are numerous saliva testing kits on the market, which can be used either in the surgery or at the sports venue (during screening) to advise athletes about the need for hydration and to test their salivary function.

In addition, the presence or absence of saliva has an important role to play in the immune response of saliva. Especially during endurance exercise, elite athletes who have a reduced saliva presence show a decrease in IgA levels, but it is unclear whether this is associated with an increase in upper respiratory tract infections [21]. Psychological stress has also been shown to decrease salivary IgA levels [22], but the relevance of this observation to immune fitness following fatiguing exercise is unclear.

1.4   The Role of Education

In common with all dental patients, it is important to emphasise the significant role that education plays in sports dentistry. We need to be able to educate our athletes from an early age about the potential problems of dental diseases and what preventative measures can be put in place. When dealing with a primarily young cohort (16–30 years), it is essential to install good habits in terms of diet, oral hygiene, and a preventative strategy. One of the problems particularly relevant to elite athletes is their availability to visit the dentist. Track and field athletes during the season are travelling the world entering various competitions and therefore are extremely difficult to tie down for a dental appointment. Sports dentists need to be aware of this and be flexible in their appointment systems to accommodate an athlete who may only be in the country for a couple of days and needs to have a dental issue resolved. This will often involve just getting the elite athlete out of pain and rearranging a suitable time for a follow-up appointment. Once free of pain, it is common for these elite athletes to forget or cancel appointments, as they are no longer uncomfortable. It is important to educate the athlete that they need further treatment before the situation deteriorates further, something which is challenging for an elite athlete who needs to catch a flight the next day to compete.

As sports dentists, we can have a positive effect on educating elite athletes during a screening session and should take every opportunity to re-iterate the preventative message whenever possible. Chapter 10 will look at screening, but suffice to say screening of soccer and rugby players in the UK is becoming more common during pre-season assessments and training; an ideal time to educate and spread the word.

1.5   The Role of Sports Dentistry

So what role can dentistry play in the world of sports medicine? The simple answer is many roles. The fundamental idea behind this book is to discuss those aspects of dentistry that have an impact on athletes from all sports and all grades of sport, and to consider how we as sports dentists can support our medical colleagues. As sports dentists we enable our colleagues in general dental and medical practices to feel confident to take an active role in the health and care of sports people and advise other health professionals on those specific areas of dental care that are particularly relevant to athletes.

The role of the sports dentist is continually evolving; initially we dealt with oro-dental trauma, then our skills spread to include emergency treatment of orofacial trauma, then prevention of injuries and most recently looking at the impact of oral health on the performance of elite athletes [19]. This book is designed to be useful to dental practitioners with a special interest in sports dentistry, as well as medical professionals who, whilst having seen dental trauma, are generally unaware of first aid measures that can make a significant difference to the long-term dental treatment of athletes. In this book we will investigate how to recognise dental trauma as a result of a sporting injury, we will consider the prevention of dental trauma, but if it should occur, how to restore those traumatised teeth, we will look at dietary advice for athletes, particularly with dental caries and tooth surface loss in mind, and consider how we can work with club doctors, physiotherapists and nutritionists.

The contents of this book form the basis of a 12-day sports dentistry programme at University College London Eastman Dental Institute that prepares general dental practitioners for dealing with athletes at all levels of sport. The programme covers all aspects of sports dentistry, including the particular problems encountered by Paralympic athletes, the role of the sports dentist with respect to banned substances that may be taken by athletes they look after, the repair of tissues following injury, i.e. muscle and bone, dealing with soft tissue injuries and the psychological implications of injuries on athletes. Teaching is a combination of seminar-based sessions and hands-on, skills-based training. Not all these issues will be dealt with in great detail in this book, but the common concerns of athletes and elite athletes in terms of sporting trauma, its prevention, dietary implications, the repair of damaged teeth, and differences between treating adults and children will be highlighted.

The London 2012 Olympic Games proved to be an inspiring and interesting opportunity to study elite athletes' oral health and previous history (see Chapter 9). The role of sports dentists in the future has been changed by the experience of those researchers at London 2012, who opened the minds of dental and medical sports practitioners as to the potentially significant role that dentists can play in elite and general sport. The interest shown worldwide in studies that emanated from those researchers has resulted in a revolution in sports dentistry and a realisation that future elite athletes need to consider their oral health along with their nutrition, cardiac physiology, fitness routines, and psychological well-being.

Elite athletes do need special consideration when it comes to dental matters and the role of prevention is paramount not just in trauma cases, but in preventing dental diseases and tooth surface loss. We need to consider dietary factors as well as the overall well-being of the athletes; screening of athletes is a very valuable way of tackling dental disease amongst a population that seems to be more prone to the ravages of dental caries, periodontal disease, and tooth erosion.

If this book inspires you to discover more about sports dentistry, please feel free to contact the editors for information on current courses/programmes. We are also happy to attend individual sporting venues, events, and clubs to advise you on how you may incorporate some of the information in this book and help your athletes achieve their ultimate goals, prevent trauma and tooth surface loss, and develop a strategy for athletes to encompass good oral health measures.

References

1 Shaw, P. (2002). Heading the ball killed England striker Jeff Astle. *Independent* (November 12).

2 Masters, J., Kessels, A., Jordan, B., Lezak, M., Troost, J. (1998). Chronic brain injury in professional soccer players. *Neurology* 51: 791–796.

3 Patton, D.A. (2016). A review of instrumented equipment to investigate head impacts in sport. *Applied Bionics and Biomechanics 2016*, Article ID 7049743, 16 pages.

4 Iverson, G.L., Gaetz, M., Lovell, M.R., Collins, M.W. (2004). Cumulative effects of concussion in amateur athletes. *Journal of Brain Injury* 18(5): 433–443.

5 Teasdale, G., Jennet, B. (1974). Assessment of coma and impaired consciousness. *The Lancet* 2(7872): 81–84.

6 Castaldi, C.R. (1986). Sports related oro-facial injuries in young athletes: a new challenge for paediatric dentists. *Paediatric Dentistry* 8(4): 311–316.

7 Blignaut, J.B., Carstens, I.L., Lombard, C.J. (1987). Injuries sustained in rugby by wearers and non-wearers of mouthguards. *British Journal of Sports Medicine* 21(2): 5–7.

8 Haug, R.H., Foss, J. (2000). Maxillofacial injuries in the paediatric patient. *Oral Surgery, Oral Medicine, Oral Pathology, Oral Radiology, Endodontics* 90(2): 126–134.

9 Hendrick, K., Farrelly, P., Jagger, R. (2008). Oro-facial injuries and mouthguard use in elite female field hockey players. *Dental Traumatology* 24(2): 189–192.

10 Huang, B., Marcenes, W., Croucher, R., Hector, M. (2009). Activities related to the occurrence of traumatic dental injuries in 15- to 18-year-olds. *Dental Traumatology* 25(1): 64–68.

11 Lambert, D.L. (2015). Splinting rationale and contemporary treatment options for luxated and avulsed permanent teeth. *General Dentistry* 63(6): 56–60.

12 Häyrinen-Immonen, R., Sane, J., Perkki, K., Malmström, M. (1990). A six-year follow-up study of sports-related dental injuries in children and adolescents. *Endodontic Dental Traumatology* 6(5): 208–212

13 Muller-Bola, M., Lupi-Pegurier, L., Pedeutoir, P., Bolla, M. (2003). Orofacial trauma and rugby in France: epidemiological survey. *Dental Traumatology* 19(4): 183–192.

14 Nysether, S. (1987). Dental injuries among Norwegian soccer players. *Community Dentistry and Oral Epidemiology* 15(3): 141–143.

15 Lindenfeld, T., Schmitt, D., Hendy, M., Mangine, R., Noyes, F. (1994). Incidence of injury in indoor soccer. *American Journal of Sports Medicine* 22: 364–371.

16 Hoff, G., Martin, T. (1986). Outdoor and indoor soccer: injuries among youth players. *American Journal of Sports Medicine* 14: 231–233.

17 Ekstrand, J., Nigg, B. (1989). Surface-related injuries in soccer. *Sports Medicine* 8: 56–62.

18 Flanders, R., Bhat, M. (1995). The incidence of oro-facial injuries in sport: a pilot study in Illinois. *Journal of the American Dental Association* 126: 491–496.

19 Needleman, I., Ashley, P., Fortune, F., et al. (2013). Oral health and impact on performance of athletes in London 2012 Olympic Games: a cross sectional study. *British Journal of Sports Medicine* 47(16): 1054–1058.

20 Andrade, R.A., Evans, P.L., Almeida, A.L., et al. (2010). Prevalence of dental trauma in Pan American Games athletes. *Dental Traumatology* 26(3): 248–253.

21 Gleeson, M., McDonald, W.A., Cripps, A.W., et al. (1995). Exercise, stress and mucosal immunity in elite swimmers. *Advances in Mucosal Immunology* 371: 571–574.

22 Jenmott, J.B., Borysenko, M., Chapman, R., et al. (1983). Academic stress, power motivation and decrease in secretion rates of saliva secretion Immunoglobulin A. *The Lancet.* 321(8339): 1400–1402.

2

Dealing with Dental Trauma: The Adult Athlete
Peter D. Fine

2.1 Introduction

In this chapter, I will consider the various injuries that occur to the hard and soft intra-oral tissues and the options that are available to treat those injuries on an immediate, mid-term, and long-term basis. Chapter 4 will deal with the repair of fractured teeth, so this chapter will consider the type of injuries commonly seen and their 'pitch-side' management. I will discuss the equipment needed to develop a pitch-side emergency dental kit, for any dentist or associated professional who may be able to give immediate relief and treatment to an injured athlete.

2.2 Classification of Injuries

There are many different ways of classifying trauma to the intra-oral dental tissues. Most divide the traumas into hard and soft tissues, or a combination of both. A systematic review of the literature was undertaken, from an epidemiological viewpoint, to evaluate the criteria used for the diagnostic classification of traumatic dental injuries [1]. The final study collection consisted of 164 articles, from 1936 to 2003, and the population sample ranged from 38 to 210,500 patients (Figure 2.1). From this, 54 distinct classification systems were identified, the most frequently used of which was the Andreasen system (32%); as regards the type of injury, the uncomplicated crown fracture was the most prominent (88.5%). Evidence suggests that there is no suitable system for establishing the diagnosis of the studied injuries that could be applied to epidemiological surveys.

An international study looked at the epidemiology of dental trauma and reported that studies demonstrated that males were more likely to experience dental trauma and that the home was the most common place for trauma to occur [2]. Sport as a cause of dental trauma was mentioned by several authors [3–7], all of whom identified maxillary central incisors as the most likely teeth to be damaged.

Due to the multi-factorial nature of traumatic dental injuries, it is difficult to classify them in a logical manner. A single traumatic episode may result in a combination of injuries to the tooth and/or supporting structures, therefore we should consider the history of the traumatic episode, the clinical signs, and the symptoms experienced by the athlete when diagnosing the problem.

2.3 Trauma to the Periodontal Ligament

Trauma to the supporting structures of the teeth (Figure 2.2) can be classified as: concussion, lateral luxation, subluxation, intrusion,

Sports Dentistry: Principles and Practice, First Edition. Edited by Peter D. Fine, Chris Louca and Albert Leung.
© 2019 John Wiley & Sons Ltd. Published 2019 by John Wiley & Sons Ltd.
Companion website: www.wiley.com/go/fine/sports_dentistry

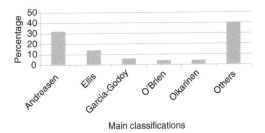

Figure 2.1 The main classification systems identified by da Costa Feliciano.

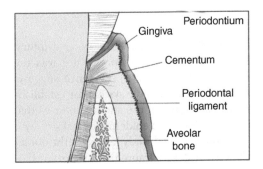

Figure 2.2 Standard arrangement of periodontal tissues.

extrusion, and avulsion. In these cases, this form of classification can be useful, as it will lead to our diagnosis and guide us to the most appropriate treatment option.

2.3.1 Concussion

Concussion is an injury to the tooth-supporting structures, but without any increased mobility or displacement of the tooth. The patient experiences some pain on percussion and there is no bleeding from the periodontal tissues. The neurovascular bundle normally remains intact, but in a few areas there is some bleeding and edema. In most cases the periodontal ligament remains undamaged. Sensitivity testing reveals a positive result, but if there is no response, this may indicate a future risk of pulp necrosis. Radiographic examination should include an occlusal view, a periapical view, and a lateral view, either from the mesial or distal direction to exclude displacement.

Follow-up appointments should be after four weeks, six to eight weeks and then one year. The vitality of the pulp should be monitored for one year. Patient advice should include the use of analgesics if required, a soft diet, and good oral hygiene practice, including chlorhexidine mouthwash.

2.3.2 Subluxation

Subluxation is an injury to the tooth's supporting structures, resulting in increased mobility of the tooth, but no displacement. There is bleeding from the gingival crevice. This type of injury is normally from a horizontal blow to the tooth (at 90° to the long axis of the tooth), which may result in damage to the neurovascular supply. In many cases there is separation of the periodontal ligament, with interstitial bleeding and edema. The tooth is tender to percussion and sensitivity testing may produce a negative response to begin with due to transient pulpal damage. The pulp should be monitored. There are no radiographic abnormalities following examination with occlusal, periapical, and lateral views.

A flexible splint should be fitted to aid patient comfort for no more than two weeks. Patient advice should include the use of analgesics if required, a soft diet, and good oral hygiene practice, including chlorhexidine mouthwash.

Follow-up appointments should be arranged after no more than two weeks to remove the splint; radiographic reviews should be conducted at two weeks, four weeks, six to eight weeks and one year.

2.3.3 Lateral Luxation

This is the displacement of a tooth other than axially. Displacement is accompanied by comminution or fracture of the surrounding bone. The etiology of the lateral luxation injury is a horizontal blow that results in a partial or total separation of the periodontal ligament, complicated by fractures to the labial and palatal/lingual bone. In most cases of lateral luxation, the apex of the tooth has been forced into the bone rendering the tooth immobile. A visual examination shows that the tooth is pointing in a labial or palatal/lingual direction. Percussion of the tooth produces a high metallic sound. Sensitivity testing will frequently give a negative response, but where a minor displacement has occurred there could be a positive response, indicating reduced risk of future pulp necrosis.

Treatment involves repositioning the tooth, normally under local anaesthetic, as soon as possible. A flexible splint should be used for approximately four weeks, in order to aid the healing of the associated bony fractures.

Radiographic examination should include an occlusal view, a periapical view, and a lateral view either from the mesial or distal direction to exclude displacement. Classically a 'halo' effect can be seen on the periapical radiograph, which, when the tooth is repositioned, disappears, indicating the tooth is back in position from an axial perspective.

Follow-up appointments for clinical and radiographic examination should be undertaken after two weeks, four weeks, six to eight weeks, six months and up to five years. Early signs of pulp necrosis should result in root canal treatment being carried out.

2.3.4 Intrusion

Of all the traumas to the supporting structures of teeth, the intrusion injury has the worst prognosis from a pulpal and periodontal health perspective. The trauma, from an axial direction upwards, drives the tooth into the alveolar bone, resulting in comminution or fracture of the alveolar socket. The tooth appears shorter than surrounding teeth, gives a high metallic sound to percussion, is immobile and produces a negative response to sensitivity testing.

Radiographic examination should include an occlusal view, a periapical view, and a lateral view either from the mesial or distal direction. The radiographs reveal a complete lack of periodontal space; the cemento-enamel junction will be apical to the surrounding teeth and possibly apical to the surrounding bony margin.

Intrusive injuries can lead to progressive root resorption, either through ankylosis or related infected resorption. Treatment is dependent on the maturity of root formation, the degree of displacement and the choice of method of repositioning (See Table 2.1).

2.3.5 Extrusion

An extrusion is the partial displacement of a tooth out of its socket, resulting in the loosening of the tooth, partial, or complete separation of the periodontal ligament, and a degree of protrusion or retrusion. Extrusive injuries result from a blow to the tooth from the apical direction. The alveolar bone is intact, and the tooth is loose, appears elongated, and is tender to percussion. Sensitivity

Table 2.1 Types of repositioning following an intrusion injury (courtesy of dentaltraumaguide.org) [8].

| | Degree of Intrusion | Repositioning | | |
		Spontaneous	Orthodontical	Surgical
Open Apex	Up to 7 mm	x		
	More than 7 mm		x	x
Closed Apex	Up to 3 mm	x		
	3–7 mm		x	x
	More than 7 mm			x

testing in mild cases can result in a positive response, indicating a reduced risk of pulp necrosis later during healing. More severe cases result in a negative response. With immature roots, pulp revascularization usually occurs, whereas in mature roots it seldom occurs.

Radiographic examination includes an occlusal view, a periapical view, and a lateral view, either from the mesial or distal direction. There is frequently an increased periodontal ligament space present.

Treatment for the extrusion injury involves cleansing the tooth root area, gently repositioning with finger pressure (using local anesthetic if needed), and splinting the tooth with a flexible splint for up to two weeks. Confirmation that the tooth is back in position correctly can be judged from the incisal edge being in line with adjacent teeth, the occlusion being satisfactory, and a normal radiographic appearance. Pulpal health should be monitored for early signs of necrosis.

The patient needs to be advised on a soft diet, regular brushing with a soft brush, chlorhexidine mouthwash, taking analgesics as needed, and the importance of regular follow-up appointments.

Follow-up appointments should be two weeks later for clinical and radiographic examination and removal of splint; further radiographic examination should be undertaken after four weeks, six to eight weeks, six months and up to five years.

2.3.6 Avulsion

Whilst relatively rare, an avulsion is the most dramatic of injuries involving the periodontal ligament – the complete loss of a tooth resulting in the severance of the neurovascular pulp supply, separation of the periodontal ligament, and exposure of the complete root surface. The signs of an avulsion should not be confused with a severe intrusion injury, where the crown of the affected tooth disappears above/below the gingival margin and is not visible to the naked eye. Radiographic

evidence plus the presentation of the tooth confirm the diagnosis. Depending on how recent the injury is, there may be either an empty socket or a coagulum present.

Routine radiographic examination should be undertaken to check the socket and any further dento-alveolar damage. Radiographs include occlusal view, a periapical view, and a lateral view either from the mesial or distal direction.

Assuming that the avulsed tooth is a permanent tooth (there is no need to replace a deciduous tooth that has been avulsed), the tooth needs to be held by the crown, washed under cool water or saline for about 10 seconds and reimplanted. The patient should be encouraged to bite into their normal occlusion to check the tooth is correctly positioned and then bite on a handkerchief or pack to hold it in place. If this is not possible, the tooth needs to be stored in a suitable medium e.g. milk, saliva in the buccal sulcus, the patient's own saliva in a pot, or Hanks balanced storage medium, which is a salt solution. The tooth can then be transported to an appropriate place for replantation.

Having checked that the tooth is in the correct position radiographically and clinically, it is splinted using a flexible splint for up to two weeks. The patient needs to be advised on a soft diet, regular brushing with a soft brush, chlorhexidine mouthwash, taking analgesics as needed, and the importance of regular follow-up appointments.

Follow-up visits should be at two weeks, for radiographic examination, splint removal, and further instructions, four weeks, six to eight weeks, six months, one year and then yearly for five years. The prognosis for replantation of avulsed teeth is dependent on several factors: the level of development of the root, how long the tooth is out of the mouth, how it has been stored, and the potential for the periodontal ligament to heal [9–12]. There has also been some research done looking at the use of chemical agents to improve the prognosis of avulsed teeth [13–15].

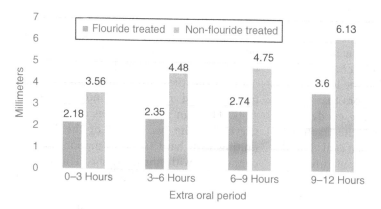

Figure 2.3 Comparison of root resorption rates with extra-oral period; three-year follow-up, following soaking in sodium fluoride [13].

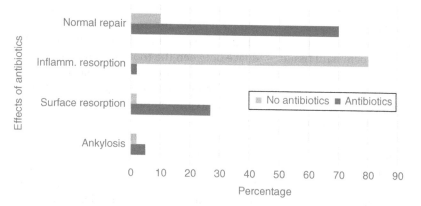

Figure 2.4 Effects of using systemic antibiotics following reimplanting avulsed adult teeth [14].

Coccia looked at the possibility of using fluoride to reduce the amount of resorption of permanent teeth following replantation [13]. After observing teeth that had been soaked for five minutes in 2% sodium fluoride, Coccia reported that, depending on how long the tooth had been out of its socket, the effects of fluoride seem to reduce the amount of resorption, over 3 years (see Figure 2.3). It is worth noting that this effect applies only to teeth where the majority of the periodontal ligament is non-viable and has been removed.

In their study, Hammarström et al., investigated the potential benefits of using both topical and systemic antibiotics following the replantation of an avulsed tooth [14].

Figure 2.4 shows that the effect of a systemic antibiotic on the periodontal ligament is to reduce inflammatory resorption, giving a greater chance for normal repair to occur.

2.4 Root Fractures

Trauma to the dentition resulting in a fracture of the root can be some of the most challenging injuries to deal with. In this section I will outline the types of root fracture commonly seen, look at the response of the tissues to root fractures, and discuss treatment options following a root fracture.

Root fractures are classified by their position on the root of the tooth: apical-third fractures, middle-third fractures, and cervical-third fractures. A correct diagnosis of the position is essential, as this is one factor may influence the type and degree of healing that we can expect [16], as well as the length and type of treatment. Other factors that influence the success of repair are age, gender, and the size of the gap between the fractured parts of the root [17]. Andreasen et al., found that a young age, (<10 years) 'immature root formation and positive pulp testing at the time of injury were significantly and positively related to both pulpal healing and hard tissue repair of the fracture' [17]. The same applied to concussion or subluxation (i.e. no displacement) of the coronal fragment compared to extrusion or lateral luxation (i.e. displacement). Furthermore, no mobility vs. mobility of the coronal fragment was significant. Girls showed more frequent hard tissue healing than boys. This relationship could possibly be explained by the fact that in this study, the girls experienced trauma at an earlier age (i.e. with more immature root formation) and their traumas were of a less severe nature. The mobility of the coronal fragment, dislocation of the coronal fragment, and diastasis between fragments (i.e. rupture or stretching of the pulp at the fracture site) also had a significant impact on repair [16]. A combination of these factors can influence the successful restoration of pulpal health, healing of the fracture, and periodontal ligament re-establishment.

Root fractures respond in four different ways: healing with calcified tissue, healing with the interposition of fibrous connective tissue, healing with the interposition of bone, and lack of healing, when granulation tissue is present in the healing site [18].

If the coronal portion of the tooth is repositioned and splinted to its original position, whilst maintaining the health of the pulp, healing will occur with calcified material in the fractured root segment. There will be dentine formation inside the pulp cavity and cementum on the root surface. Gradually the dentine will obliterate the pulp in the apical portion.

If the coronal and apical segments cannot be repositioned accurately, interposition of blood clots in the fracture site will occur. As healing progresses, granulation tissue originating from the pulp or periodontal tissue occupies and proliferates into the blood clots. This can result in areas of resorption preventing the two halves of the fracture uniting with hard tissue formation, instead connecting with fibrous tissue. This can be recognised radiographically as rounded edges of the fracture site.

Healing with interposition of bone and connective tissue occurs when the root fracture occurs in early development of the tooth. If the fracture is healed by the interposition of connective tissue only the coronal aspect of the tooth will continue to erupt; consequently bone will infill the space between the tooth fragments.

If the pulpal tissues becomes necrotic there will be an interposition of granulation tissue. In order to prevent bone loss and resorption of the root, it is necessary to remove the necrotic pulp and undertake endodontic treatment (see Chapter 5).

The aetiology of root fracture is from a blow to the tooth, resulting in the tissues of the root fracturing. This leads to damage to the neurovascular supply of the tooth at the fracture site, with the apical segment remaining intact. There is also some damage to the periodontal ligament at the fracture site and displacement of the segments. As a result of a root fracture, the coronal segment may be loose or even displaced, the crown of the tooth will have a transient discolouration, there will be bleeding from the gingival crevice, and the tooth will be tender to percussion. Initial sensitivity may be negative due to transient or permanent nerve damage. Careful monitoring is essential. Radiographic examination should include occlusal and periapical views. Occlusal radiographs are ideal for locating middle- or apical-third fractures, whereas the periapical, bisecting angle exposure is needed for cervical-third fractures.

Treatment of root fractures depends to a certain extent on their diagnosis. With apical- and middle-third fractures, the tooth is cleaned with saline, repositioned by finger pressure, acid etched and composite applied to secure the flexible metal splint. This should be left in place for four weeks. A cervical-third fracture should be treated in the same way, but the splint should be in place for up to four months. The tooth needs to be monitored radiographically and clinically at four weeks, six to eight weeks, four months, one year and then every year for at least five years; any signs of pulp necrosis need to be treated with root canal therapy.

2.5   Splinting Techniques

Dental splints can be divided into those for occlusal purposes, i.e. Michigan splint, those used for orthodontic reasons, and those splints used following trauma. In this section, I will deal primarily with those splints that we construct following a traumatic incident to the dentition. The main purpose of the splint is to provide support for traumatized teeth during the initial healing phase. There is a huge variety of materials that are available for splinting teeth, but the ideal splinting material should possess the following properties:

- Quick and easy to construct
- Allows physiological mobility
- Easy to clean
- Passive
- Doesn't cause gingival damage
- Comfortable
- Durable
- Relatively easy to remove
- No occlusal interference.

The materials that we use on a routine basis are acid etch composite (AEC), AEC and wire, milk bottle top and zinc oxide/eugenol cement, orthodontic brackets and wire, mesh splint, kevlar thread, and titanium. Acid etch composite is relatively easy to use, cheap, and available. The tooth/teeth need to be repositioned, cleaned, and dried as well as possible,

and then either flowable or regular composite applied to the labial surface of the damaged teeth and light-cured. This is particularly helpful in an emergency situation at the local sports club (see Chapter 11).

A slightly more sophisticated splint could be made by bending a soft round wire, which can then be passively bonded to the damaged teeth by composite. The wire helps to give support to the teeth, whilst using less composite, which means the splint is more comfortable to wear, easier to remove and still allows for some physiological movement to occur. It is important that the wire is passive when in place so as not to act as an orthodontic appliance. If only one tooth is affected, splinting of that tooth and one tooth either side of it is usually sufficient. For example if a central incisor suffers a luxation injury and splinting is recommended, the splint should go from the lateral incisor on the same side, to the central incisor on the other side.

A traditional method of splinting luxated teeth, particularly pitch-side, was to use a silver milk bottle top. Having cleaned and repositioned the luxated tooth/teeth, the metal would be cut to shape, molded around the teeth, and cemented in place with zinc phosphate cement until the patient could attend the surgery and have a more sophisticated splint fitted. This worked well, but has some limitations, including being difficult to remove, traumatic to the soft tissues, interfering with the occlusion, and unsightly.

If a luxation injury occurs to teeth that are undergoing orthodontic treatment with fixed bands in place, these bands can act as an effective splint, once the tooth/teeth have been repositioned. Referral to the orthodontic specialist following emergency repair of orthodontic appliances is recommended to ensure that forces detrimental to tooth movement have not been inadvertently introduced.

A mesh splint material, originally designed for splinting periodontally involved teeth can be used very successfully to splint luxated teeth. Having repositioned the teeth, this fine mesh is cut to length and thickness with scissors, bent into an arch shape by finger pressure, and cemented in place with flowable composite. This material is easy to use, easy to remove, soft enough to not cause any periodontal damage, and cheap to purchase (see Figure 2.5). Cleaning the material can be a little difficult, but generally speaking it works very well.

Kevlar thread is a material more associated with fishing or sewing. Following repositioning of luxated teeth, the thread is cut to length and twisted in order to incorporate several thicknesses and cemented with composite. It is manufactured in three thicknesses, namely, 0.0081, 0.0140, and 0.0255 inches. As the thread gets thicker so its strength increases (see Figure 2.6). Kevlar thread provides a passive splint that is easy to remove, comfortable to wear, and aesthetically acceptable. The downside is it is a little difficult to fabricate the splint as the material is not at all rigid.

The titanium trauma splint is much more advanced. This product has been recognised as having all the qualities required of a splinting material. It is easy to handle, as it can be bent by hand, so there is no need for wire-bending equipment; it is flexible enough, easy to remove and clean up; if positioned correctly does not interfere with the gingival tissues, is relatively aesthetic, and is comfortable for the patient (see Figure 2.7). The titanium trauma splint comes in two lengths: 52 mm and 100 mm, but can be cut to size. Having repositioned the luxated tooth/teeth, they are cleaned with pumice, etched, and bond is applied. The pre-shaped splint is then positioned on the labial surfaces of the affected teeth and set in place with composite. Polishing of the composite for comfort completes the procedure. The only disadvantage of this material is the cost.

This is by no means an exhaustive list of splinting materials, but it should be emphasised that with all splinting materials, the ease of use and removal, the aesthetics, the comfort, the cost, the passivity, the cleanability, and the provision of support, while allowing physiological movement of the tooth, are all essential. I have mentioned the need for the splint to be flexible, which means that we don't want to use a material that is

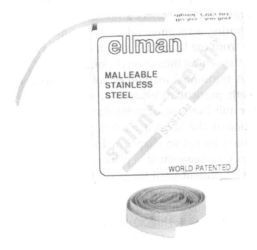

Figure 2.5 Ellman mesh splint.

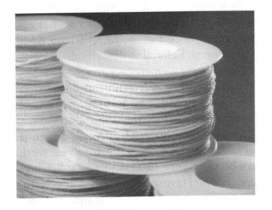

Figure 2.6 **Kevlar thread.**

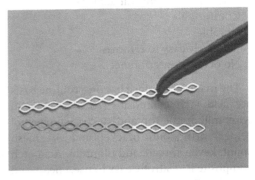

Figure 2.7 Titanium trauma splint (Medartis AG, Basel, Switzerland).

too rigid for luxation injuries. The maximum diameter of the material used should be 0.4 mm [13]. The exception to using a flexible splint is when dealing with a root fracture. In this instance a rigid splint should be used, such as a rectangular orthodontic wire, but otherwise similar principles apply.

2.6 Ankylosis

Dentoalveolar ankylosis is a serious complication of the periodontal ligament following trauma to the dentition. Quite simply, ankylosis is a fusion of the tooth to the alveolar bone, which results in progressive resorption of the root surface, which is replaced by bone (replacement resorption). In the patient that is still growing, ankylosis can result in reduced growth of the alveolar process. It is important to consider ankylosis in this chapter on dealing with dental trauma as sporting injuries can result in avulsions and intrusion injuries, which can be particularly liable to ankylosis. Patients/parents need to be warned about this very real possibility and advised about the guarded long-term prognosis for these teeth.

In the case of intrusion and avulsion injuries, we have discussed the need for splinting the teeth. One of the fundamental aspects of these trauma splints is to allow physiological movement of the tooth during healing, and so the splint needs to be removed after 28 days. Prolonged use of a splint can result in ankylosis of the tooth, which may be transient unless the injury to the cementum is extensive. This transient ankylosis can commence two to three weeks after reimplanting the avulsed tooth. The healing processes are initiated from the bone on the alveolar side of the periodontal ligament or from adjacent bone marrow resulting in ankylosis between socket wall and root surface. Ankylosis is strongly related to the extent of damage to the periodontal ligament on the root surface during the extra-alveolar period. Fractures of the alveolar bone adjacent to the replantation site are more prone to ankylosis.

Ankylosis can be detected both clinically and radiographically. Clinical signs include the use of percussion sounds and the degree of mobility in a labial/lingual direction. The ankylosed tooth produces a characteristically high-pitched sound when percussed, compared to adjacent healthy teeth. Studies using digital sound-wave analysis have shown that the sound emitted by an ankylosed tooth when it is percussed has a significantly higher proportion of the sound energy in the higher frequency bands [19]. Over many years, a variety of quantitative methods for measuring tooth mobility have been developed [20]. These have proved to be somewhat unreliable in clinical use. However, the introduction of Periotest (Siemans, Germany) has proved to be quite reliable in the diagnosis of ankylosed compared to intact incisors, but a low Periotest score alone should not be considered diagnostic for ankylosis.

Radiographic examination is considered to be of limited value in the early detection of ankylosis due to the two-dimensional nature of the radiograph. The initial location for ankylosis is in the labial and lingual/palatal aspects of the tooth, making radiographic detection more difficult [21,22].

Combined clinical, radiographic, and mobility findings indicate that healing after replantation can be divided into the following modalities:

1) Normal healing with slightly increased or normal mobility values and no radiographic sign of progressive root resorption.
2) Permanent replacement resorption with lowered mobility values and radiographic signs of replacement resorption. Decreased mobility values indicate that ankylosis is usually evident five weeks after replantation. At the same time, it was possible to diagnose the ankylosis by the percussion test. Radiographic examination first reveals ankylosis eight weeks after replantation.
3) Transient replacement resorption (not previously described) with lowered mobility values, which later become

normal. Radiographic signs of a transient replacement resorption are present in some cases.

4) Inflammatory resorption with increased mobility values and radiographic signs of inflammatory root resorption. Mobility values tend to become normal when inflammation subsides as a result of root canal treatment.

The storage of the avulsed tooth is recognised as being critical to the success or otherwise of the replantation procedure. Several different media have been tried to determine which is most appropriate. Of course the best

treatment is immediate replantation of the avulsed tooth, which is the where the sports dentist being on site at sporting events can prove to be most useful. The principle is to try and preserve the viable cells within the periodontal ligament. If a solution needs to be used to store the tooth, milk with a pH of 6.5–6.8 and osmolarity of 230–270 mOsm/kg is most compatible with long-term cell survival [24–26]. Saliva is also a suitable medium, but tap water, which has hypotonic properties, can be as damaging as storing the tooth dry [27]. Various media have been tried as suitable storage with mixed success [28] (see Figures 2.8–2.10).

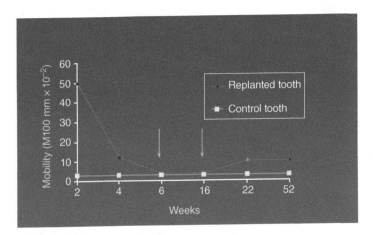

Figure 2.8 Graph of transient ankylosis following replantation [23].

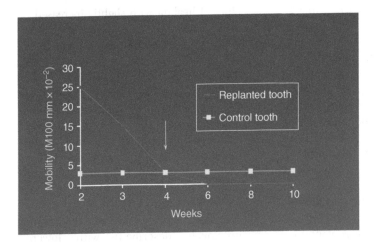

Figure 2.9 Graph of ankylosis following replantation [23].

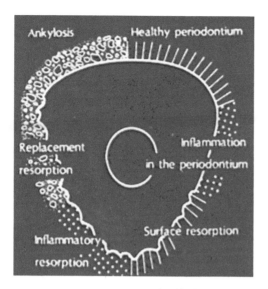

Figure 2.10 The most common periodontal repair patterns observed during replantation [14].

2.7 Soft Tissue Injuries

Soft tissue injuries commonly occur during sport, particularly contact sports like hockey (Figure 2.11) [29]. In this study it was shown that 68% of the cohort of English, female, field hockey players received oro-facial trauma, and of those, 87.3% of the injuries were soft tissue injuries.

In martial arts sports like taekwondo, the prevalence of soft tissue injuries can be quite high compared to other types of injury [30]. Of the 54 subjects (19.7%) suffering soft tissue injuries, 44 were female (81.5%), while only 10 were male (18.5%), of which 40 (74.1%) were taekwondo practitioners and 14 (25.9%) were boxers.

Soft tissue injuries can be divided into four categories: contusion, abrasion, laceration, and penetrating wound. The treatment of the soft tissue trauma will depend on its diagnosis and cause. Contusions are soft tissue injuries that cause swelling and pain, and limit the range of movement near the injury (Figure 2.12). Torn blood vessels may cause bluish discoloration. The injury may feel weak and stiff. Sometimes a pool of blood collects within damaged tissue, forming a

lump over the injury (haematoma). Examples of trauma are a cut or a blow to the soft tissues of the lip, gingivae, or cheek. The injury causes capillaries to burst. The blood gets trapped below the skin's surface, which causes a bruise. The contusion can be treated by applying ice on a regular basis, which will reduce the swelling and bruising by constricting the capillaries.

Abrasion injuries most commonly occur when exposed skin comes into moving contact with a rough surface, causing a grinding or rubbing away of the upper layers of the epidermis (Figure 2.13). Conventional treatment of abrasions includes cleaning the wound with mild soap and water or a mild antiseptic wash, and then applying an antiseptic ointment. Applying ice will also help to reduce swelling and aid comfort.

A laceration is a wound that is produced by the tearing of soft body tissue (Figure 2.14). This type of wound is often irregular and jagged. A laceration wound is often contaminated with bacteria and debris from whatever object caused the cut. In the oro-facial area, contamination intra-orally can occur when the laceration is on the skin and penetrates through to the intra-oral area. This may be due to a blow to the face from a hockey stick, a cricket ball or a collision with another player. It may also be caused by an incorrectly shaped and finished mouthguard piecing the oral soft tissue following a blow. Good wound cleansing is important and sutures may be required. If the wound extends beyond the vermillion border of the lip, it may be appropriate to enlist the help of a plastic surgeon for the definitive repair, unless the dentist is skilled in that field.

Penetrating wounds occur when a foreign body has penetrated the dermis and remained in situ (Figure 2.15). It is frequently difficult to identify the object, particularly if presentation of the wound is some time after the trauma. A radiograph can be helpful to identify foreign bodies below the surface. The wound needs to be cleaned and the removal of the object arranged before satisfactory healing can be expected. A common penetrating wound

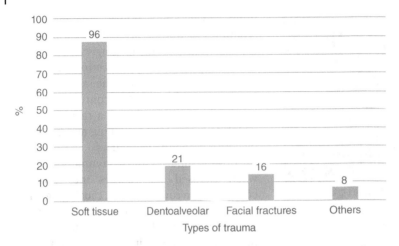

Figure 2.11 Distribution of dental trauma in female field hockey players.

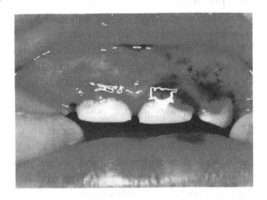

Figure 2.12 Contusion of gingival tissues.

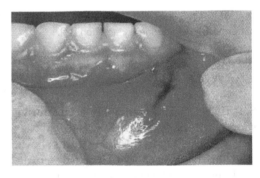

Figure 2.14 Laceration of lower lip.

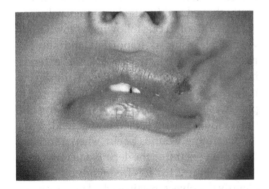

Figure 2.13 Abrasion of upper lip.

occurs when someone's front teeth are in collision with an opponent and fracture, leaving the fractured segment embedded in the chin, lip or skull of the player.

With intra-oral soft tissue traumas, it is worth considering putting the patient on antibiotics for three to five days. Sutures can be removed after about five days (unless self-dissolving sutures are used). A soft diet is to be encouraged, as is good oral hygiene procedures, including the use of a chlorhexidine mouthwash.

2.8 Developing an Emergency Dental Kit

When attending sporting events, either professional or amateur, it is unlikely that a fully equipped dental suite will be available for the sports dentist to treat field-of-play emergencies. Therefore, it is likely that a

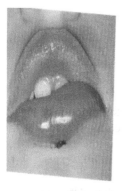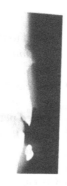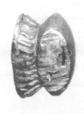

Figure 2.15 Penetrating wound from an air gun pellet.

small emergency kit, developed by the sports dentist, will be a useful adjunct to caring for injured athletes. The essence of the kit is that it should be small, portable, light to carry, and have all the necessary equipment contained in the bag to deal with field-of-play dental injuries. At many sporting events the physiotherapy table will have to be used as a dental chair, but where this is not an option any chair to seat the athlete can to be used. In Chapter 11, we shall deal with setting up dental facilities at sporting events, so I will not investigate that aspect here.

The field-of-play kit is designed to deal with the immediate effect of the trauma, prior to either taking the athlete to the dental surgery for more definitive treatment or referring to a local hospital if facial fractures are suspected, getting the athlete back onto the field of play, if safe to do so, and advising the medical team about the athletes suitability to continue.

The kit should contain:

- Headlight (walker's LED headlights are suitable)
- Sterile gloves for the dentist
- Face mask (if required)
- Dental mirror, tweezers, probe, periodontal probe, flat plastic, excavator (disposable)
- Local anaesthetic syringe and cartridges (disposable)
- Etch and bond (all-in-one)
- Composite restorative material
- Flowable composite restorative material
- Glass ionomer restorative material
- Cordless light curing machine
- Sterile gauze, cotton wool rolls, and pressure packs
- Saline solution
- Suture set and suture material
- Steri-strips
- Tooth splinting material (orthodontic wire, titanium trauma splint etc.)
- Wire-bending tool
- Note pad and camera
- Sharps box
- Kit bag to carry on.

The use of a note pad and camera could be invaluable if the treatment provided by the sports dentist is ever questioned at a later date. Contemporaneous notes and photographs may be invaluable if the treatment provided at the pitch side is disputed. I have included Steri-strips within the emergency kit as these can be helpful if there is a facial laceration that the sports dentist does not feel competent or confident enough to suture, and would prefer to refer to a plastic surgeon. The wound can be temporarily closed prior to referral to the correct specialist. The use of disposable instruments is not essential, but desirable, as there may not be appropriate sterilising facilities on-site. The sports dentist could of course take instruments back to their surgery to undergo correct disinfection, sterilization, and packaging.

References

1 Da Costa Feliciano, K., de Franca Caldes, A. (2006). A systematic review of the diagnostic classification of traumatic dental injuries. *Dental Traumatology* 22(2): 71–76.

2 Bastone, E.B., Freer, T.J., McNamara, J.R. (2000). Epidemiology of dental trauma: a review of the literature. *Australian Dental Journal* 45(1): 2–9.

3 Liew, V.P., Daly, C.G. (1986). anterior dental traumatology treated after hours in Newcastle, Australia. *Community Dental Epidemiology* 14: 362–366.

4 Martin, I.G., Daly, C.G., Liew, V.P. (1990). After hours treatment of dental trauma in Newcastle and Western Sydney: a four year study. *Australian Dental Journal* 35: 27–31.

5 Caliskan, M.K., Turkum, M. (1995). Clinical investigation of traumatic of permanent incisors in Izmir, Turkey. *Endodontic Dental Traumatology* 11: 210–213.

6 Stockwell, A.J. (1988). Incidence of dental trauma in Western Australian Schools Dental Service. *Community Dental Oral Epidemiology* 16: 294–298.

7 Perez, R., Berkowitz, R., McIlveen, L., Forrester, D. (1991). Dental Trauma in Children Survey. *Endodontic Dental Traumatology* 7: 212–213.

8 Andreasen, J., Bakland, L., Matras, R., Andreasen, F. (2006). Traumatic intrusion of permanent teeth. Part 1. An epidemiological study of 216 intruded permanent teeth. *Dental Traumatology* 22(20): 83–89.

9 Andreasen, J., Borum, M., Jacobson, H., Andreasen, F. (1995). Replantation of 400 avulsed permanent incisors. I. Diagnosis of healing complications. *Endodontic Dental Traumatology* 11: 51–58.

10 Andreasen, J., Borum, M., Jacobson, H., Andreasen, F. (1995). Replantation of 400 avulsed permanent incisors. II. Factors related to pulpal healing. *Endodontic Dental Traumatology* 11: 59–68.

11 Andreasen, J., Borum, M., Jacobson, H., Andreasen, F. (1995). Replantation of 400 avulsed permanent incisors. III. Factors related to root growth after replantation. *Endodontic Dental Traumatology* 11: 69–75.

12 Andreasen, J., Borum, M., Jacobson, H., Andreasen, F. (1995). Replantation of 400 avulsed permanent incisors. IV. Factors related to periodontal ligament healing. *Endodontic Dental Traumatology* 11: 76–89.

13 Coccia, C.T. (1980). A clinical investigation of root resorption rates in reimplanted young permanent incisors: a five-year study. *Journal of Endodontics* 6(1): 413–420.

14 Hammarström, L., Blomlöf, L., Feiglin, B., Andersson, L., Lindskog, S. (1986). Replantation of teeth and antibiotic treatment. *Endodontic Dental Traumatology* 2(2): 51–57.

15 Cvek, M., Cleaton-Jones, P., Austin, J., et al. (1980). Effects of topical application of doxycycline on pulp revascularization and periodontal healing in re-implanted monkey incisors. *Dental Traumatology* 6(4): 170–176.

16 Kwan, S.C., Johnson, J.D., Cohenca, N. (2012). The effect of splint material and thickness on tooth mobility after extraction and replantation using a human cadaveric model. *Dental Traumatology* 28: 277–281.

17 Andreasen, J., Andreasen, F., Megare, I., Cvek, M. (2004). Healing of 400 intra-alveolar root fractures. 1. Effect of pre-injury and injury factors such as sex, age, stage of root development, fracture type, location of fracture and severity of dislocation. *Dental Traumatology* 20(4): 192–202.

18 Tsukiboshi, M. (2000). *Treatment Planning for Traumatized Teeth*. Quintessence Publishing.

19 Campbell, K.M., Casas, M.J., Kenny, D.J., Chau, T. (2005). Diagnosis of ankylosis in permanent incisors by expert ratings; periotest and digital sound wave analysis. *Dental Traumatology* 21(4): 206–212.

20 Yankell, S. (1988). Review of methods of measuring tooth mobility. *Compendium Supplement* 9(12): S428–S432.

21 Andersson, L. (1988). Dentoalveola ankyloses and associated root resorption in replanted teeth: Experimental and clinical studies in monkeys and man. *Swedish Dental Journal Supplement* 56: 1–57.

22 Stenvik, A., Beyer-Olsen, E.M., Abyholm, F., Hannaes, H.R., Gerner, N.W. (1990). Validity of the radiographic assessment of anylosis: evaluation of lomg term reactions in 10 monkey incisors. *Acta Odontologica Scandinivica* 48(4): 265–269.

23 Andreasen J. (1975). The effects of splinting upon periodontal healing after replantation of permanent incisors in monkeys. *Acta Odontologica Scandinivica* 33(6): 313–323.

24 Lindskoc, S., Blomlof, L. (1982). Influence of osmolality and composition of some storage media on human periodontal ligament cells. *Acta Odontologica Scandinivica* 40: 435–441.

25 Blomlof, L., Lindskog, S., Hammarström, L. (1981). Periodontal healing of exarticulated teeth stored in milk or saliva. *Scandinavian Journal of Dental Research* 89: 251–259.

26 Blomlof, I., Otteskog P. (1980). Viability of human periodontal ligament cells after storage in milk or saliva. *Scandinavian Journal of Dental Research* 88: 436–440.

27 Blomlof, L. (1981). Milk and saliva as possible storage media for traumatically exarticulated teeth prior to replantation. *Swedish Dental Journal Supplement* 8: 1–26.

28 Hammarström, L., Blomlöf, L., Feigli, B., Lindskog, S. (1986). Tooth avulsion and replantation: a review. *Endodontic Dental Traumatology* 2: 1–8.

29 Hendrick, K., Farrelly, P., Jagger, R. (2008). Oro-facial injuries and mouthguard use in elite female field hockey players. *Dental Traumatology* 24: 189–192.

30 Tulunoglu, I., Ozbek, M. (2006). Oral trauma, mouthguard awareness, and use in two contact sports in Turkey. *Dental Traumatology* 22(5): 242–246.

3

Dealing with Sporting Dental Trauma in Paediatric Patients
Paul Ashley

3.1 Introduction

Loss or damage to teeth in children is painful and disfiguring. It will have long-term effects on the growth and development of the mouth, and will impact on a young person's appearance and general quality of life. Management is expensive, time consuming, and lifelong, and in a child or adolescent may need multidisciplinary input from specialist paediatric dentists and orthodontists.

Ideally, sport-related dental trauma is prevented by simple interventions, such as mouthguards; this is dealt elsewhere in this book and in this chapter. However, dental trauma is often unavoidable, particularly in sport, therefore understanding how to manage this trauma when it happens is crucial. Emergency care provided at the time of an injury can profoundly affect the prognosis. This initial emergency management will have to be provided by those on the scene of the trauma. In the case of sport-related dental trauma, this could include family members, coaches, emergency doctors, or other non-dental professionals.

This chapter aims to outline the emergency management of dental trauma with an emphasis on the treatment that should be provided at or around the time of the injury. It will focus on trauma to the permanent dentition of older children and adolescents, as younger children who still have significant numbers of primary teeth are unlikely to be playing competitive sport (though trauma to primary teeth will be discussed briefly). Emergency management will be described so that where possible it could be provided by whoever is available at the time of the injury. Then an overview of the treatment provided subsequently by the dental professional will be given. A more detailed description of subsequent dental treatment is outside of the scope of this chapter; for more detailed information on dental management, guidance provided by the International Association of Dental Traumatology (IADT) is an excellent place to start [1]. This chapter will also not consider management of facial fractures; the focus is on damage to the teeth.

3.2 Dental Trauma: Children vs. Adults

Why is dental trauma in children and adolescents different to trauma in adults? There are two main reasons why adolescents and young adults present a more complex management challenge compared to adults. The first is around behaviour management and age. This group may be unable to cope with complex dental treatment due to their age and stage of psychological development. Significant dental trauma can require multiple visits and invasive dental procedures. Young or anxious

Sports Dentistry: Principles and Practice, First Edition. Edited by Peter D. Fine, Chris Louca and Albert Leung.
© 2019 John Wiley & Sons Ltd. Published 2019 by John Wiley & Sons Ltd.
Companion website: www.wiley.com/go/fine/sports_dentistry

children may simply be unable to cope with this. As a result, they may need referral to a specialist dental setting with experience in managing behaviour in this age group. This will further complicate delivery of effective emergency management.

The other difference between children and adults with regard to dental trauma is related to growth and development – principally dental development and growth of the alveolar bone. This group will not have reached physical maturity, which limits the types of treatment that can be provided. Continuing growth means that some of the principles for managing trauma in adults do not apply, and that for some types of trauma a different set of problems present themselves.

3.3 Dental Development and Trauma

As teeth grow, the tooth root lengthens and the walls thicken until the root is fully developed, leaving only a narrow orifice at the end of the root through which the blood vessels and nerves can communicate with the dental pulp. With regard to dental trauma, the important teeth to consider are the front permanent incisor teeth; these teeth do not complete development until approximately 10–11 years of age [2]. Understanding the stage of root development when a trauma occurs is important because:

1) If root development stops before it is complete as a result of dental trauma (e.g. crown fracture leading to loss of pulp vitality) then this leaves a tooth root that is thin, prone to damage, and more difficult to treat using conventional methods.
2) If the blood supply into the tooth is disrupted (e.g. following avulsion), an immature root with a wide-open root end will be more likely to regain this blood supply following the injury. A tooth with a mature root and very narrow root end is much less likely to regain the blood supply and therefore more likely to become non-vital following an injury.

3.4 Alveolar Bone Growth and Trauma

As we grow and mature physically, the teeth are not the only structures in the mouth that change. The alveolar bone and jaws are also in development. During development, alveolar bone grows horizontally and vertically. This continues right through adolescence and does not stop until skeletal growth is complete. This growth is important when considering the prognosis of periodontal ligament injuries. If the periodontal ligament surrounding the tooth root is damaged, the tooth can become fused (ankylosed) to the bone. In adults, this is not usually an issue, but in a developing adolescent it can cause significant problems. Normally the tooth will be 'carried' with the alveolar bone as it grows vertically; however, in cases of ankylosis it appears to sink into the gum over time as the alveolar bone grows past it. This is called infraocclusion. This process cannot be reversed and if it is not managed, will result in very poor aesthetics of the affected area. The continuing growth of the alveolar bone also means that dental implants are not an option for tooth replacement in this group. This can be an issue if a tooth is lost at a young age. Teeth are required to maintain alveolar bone height and thickness. If they are lost and not replaced this can result in atrophy of the alveolus which can make subsequent dental implant placement (once growth is complete) difficult to carry out.

Finally, it's worth noting that adolescents are often having orthodontic treatment; this is commonly carried out in this age group as it is thought that the continuing skeletal growth will support tooth movement. This can influence treatment planning, as it may be possible to remove a traumatised tooth with a poor long-term prognosis and guide the development of the other teeth to fill the resulting gap. This will then remove the need for long-term restoration of the space. Dental trauma may also affect the delivery of orthodontics, and traumatised teeth may be at greater risk of root resorption if they are moved orthodontically. Orthodontics is possible in a mouth with traumatised teeth, but should be carried out with caution.

3.5   Epidemiology

Exact figures for the epidemiology of trauma in children vary (available data on prevalence ranges from 6–59 %) and are complicated by differences in the way in which trauma is measured or classified. Nevertheless, it is generally accepted that approximately one-third of all pre-schoolers will have trauma affecting their primary teeth and one-quarter of adolescents and adults will have trauma affecting their adult teeth at least once during their life [3].

In the adolescent and adult group, sport-related activities are the most common cause for dental trauma; this appears to be more likely in physically active individuals. However, data for the prevalence of trauma in different sports in a child or adolescent group is unavailable. A greater preponderance of traumatic dental injuries in males relative to females is commonly described, though this difference seems to be in decline. Anterior teeth (particularly upper front teeth) are most commonly affected by dental trauma, with crown fractures being the most common injuries and usually only one tooth affected. Individuals who have had trauma previously may be more likely to experience trauma again.

3.6   Preventing Trauma

Mouthguards are covered at length elsewhere in this book; however, it is worthwhile remembering that in this group, mouthguards will need to take account of the growth of the child and will need replacing at regular intervals to ensure they fit. They may also be complicated to fabricate if orthodontic treatment is being provided with a fixed appliance. This will need input from a dentist or orthodontist, but orthodontics should not be a barrier to playing sport safely with an effective mouthguard.

One other area of trauma prevention that is perhaps unique to this group is the risk presented by a large incisal overjet (horizontal space between the tip of the front teeth and the labial surface of the lower incisor teeth [Figure 3.1]). Prominent front teeth are at greater risk of trauma because of their position; they will be one of the first things to be traumatised in the event of any sort of impact. An incisal overjet of greater than 6 mm can double or even triple the risk of trauma [4]. Children with large overjets taking part in sport should therefore consider having early orthodontic intervention to reduce the overjet (as well using mouthguards).

Finally, wisdom teeth develop and erupt in the young adult [2], usually starting to appear between 16 and 17 years of age. Up until this point, they are growing and developing in the bones of the jaw, in the case of lower wisdom teeth they are located at the angle of the mandible. There is some evidence to suggest that unerupted lower wisdom teeth could be

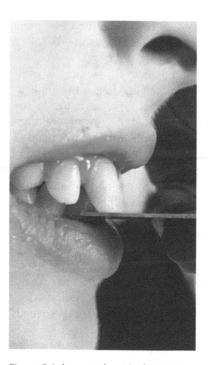

Figure 3.1 Increased overjet being measured.

linked with an increased risk of fracture – the unerupted tooth near the angle of the mandible reduces the amount of bone and hence the strength of the bone [5]. Specific guidance does not exist; however, it might be wise to consider screening for this – particularly in young athletes where a blow to the mandible is likely.

3.7 Emergency Management of Dental Trauma

The aim of this section is to give an overview of management with a focus on what should be done at the time of the injury, where dental input may not be available; however, it is important to note that dental management of dental trauma is best provided by a dentist [6]. Ideally, any sporting complex, tournament, league etc. should have a system where rapid access to dental advice or treatment can be provided. Failing that, clear instructions on how to manage common dental injuries (in particular avulsion) should be available.

With regard to trauma in the developing dentition, it is helpful to differentiate between injuries to the hard tissues (e.g. enamel, dentine) and injuries to the supportive periodontal ligament (Figure 3.2), as the implications of the different types of injury in the developing dentition and growing child are significant. Young athletes may experience a combination of both injuries.

Injuries to the dental hard tissues will cause discomfort, aesthetic concerns and ultimately may lead to loss of pulp vitality. Teeth with non-vital pulps are weaker, even following treatment. Loss of pulp vitality in a developing tooth will also stop root formation, further complicating treatment and weakening the tooth. However, therapies to manage injuries to dental hard tissues can be effective, and overall the prognosis for these teeth is not necessarily terminal.

Injuries to the periodontal ligament are difficult to treat, with eventual loss of the

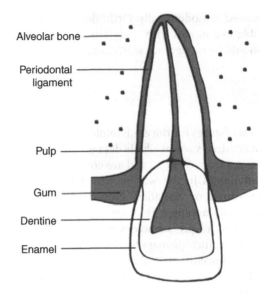

Figure 3.2 Diagram of an upper permanent incisor tooth illustrating key structures.

tooth more likely. Problems might include fusion of the tooth to the bone (ankylosis) with subsequent 'sinking' of the tooth into the jaw as the alveolar bone develops (infraocclusion), or resorption of the tooth root by the immune system, leading to eventual early tooth loss.

Whatever the injury, the key to good initial management is an accurate initial assessment. The rest of this section assumes that more significant medical issues such as concussion have been managed.

3.7.1 Assessment

Early effective management of dental trauma can have a profound influence on the outcome. So, as long as it is safe for the individual, some sort of timely dental assessment can make a big difference. Key components of any dental assessment are the soft tissues and the teeth. When considering the teeth we should think about the dental hard tissues (is the tooth intact or broken) and the periodontal ligament (is the tooth in the correct place and firm or is it loose). Any assessment will consist of a history and a visual examination.

History:

1) Was there a period of unconsciousness? Possibly the most important question you need to ask. Clearly, early management of trauma is important and will greatly improve the prognosis. But management of a concussion is more important.

2) What is the medical history (including tetanus vaccination)? Medical conditions that might influence trauma management are rare and outside of the scope of this book. Nevertheless, it is important to take a brief medical history if the patient is unknown to you. Tetanus status is important if the soft tissues have been abraded or lacerated or if a tooth needs replanting in the mouth. Uncertainty around tetanus status shouldn't stop you from replanting a tooth, but should be followed up later with a medical professional

3) Trauma history. Specifically where did it happen, when did it happen and how did it happen. A brief trauma history is important if you did not witness the traumatic event as it may give you some clues as to the type of injury. In particular, this can help you locate any tooth fragments or whole teeth if they are missing. If the tooth is dislodged, either completely or in part, it is important to identify where the missing piece has gone. If it is not located then it could be embedded in the soft tissue or possibly inhaled or swallowed. If inhaled then this may require further investigation, the decision as to whether a chest x-ray is required to locate any missing fragment will need to be made by a physician familiar with this sort of presentation, e.g. an attending physician at an accident and emergency department. If the piece is located then this can be stored in water or saline and taken to any subsequent dental visit, as in some cases reattachment of the fragment may be possible.

Visual assessment:

1) Clean the face and teeth with water. Identify any external abrasions that may need to be cleaned more thoroughly or sutured. Palpate the facial bones to check for any facial fractures.

2) Assess intra-oral soft tissue injuries. Are there any intra-oral lacerations, is any of the tooth root or alveolar bone exposed?

3) Assess the bite, i.e. do the teeth meet together normally? If they don't this could be a sign of tooth displacement or even of a facial fracture.

4) Look at the teeth – are any of them damaged? Are any of them loose? Are all the teeth and pieces of teeth accounted for?

Any verbal and visual assessment should be thorough enough to support good follow-on care. However, in the case of an avulsed tooth, every minute the tooth is out of the mouth the prognosis for the tooth worsens. Therefore, the verbal and visual assessment need to be efficient as well.

3.7.2 General Management

Once a verbal and visual assessment has been carried out, management can be planned. General management for any dental trauma is reassurance, soft diet, analgesics, as required, and chlorhexidine mouth rinse or gel (for approximately a week). Use of chlorhexidine helps keep the surrounding intra-oral gingivae and soft tissues clean immediately following a dental injury when tooth brushing might be difficult. Older children can use a mouthrinse, younger children who may have difficulty with rinsing and spitting should use the gel applied using a swab or similar. After this 'ringside' management has been completed, the individual should be referred on to a dentist for a fuller assessment and treatment. Further diagnostic tests that a dentist might commonly use are radiographs and sensibility tests such as thermal sensitivity or electric pulp tests. Traumatised teeth can cause problems several years after the initial injury, so long-term follow up is an important part of any management strategy.

3.8   Management of Soft Tissue Injuries

Any abrasions or lacerations should be inspected for contamination and may require cleaning and taping shut (if extra-oral). Intra-oral lacerations are difficult to manage in this way so may require further specialist treatment by an oral surgeon, paediatric dentist or other appropriate specialist. As a short-term measure, use of a swab or gauze held in the mouth may help. Intra-oral lacerations, if minor, can be left, but significant lacerations may require suturing. Gingival lacerations or displacement resulting in exposed tooth root or alveolar bone should be carefully repositioned and sutured into place. Any lip lacerations involving the vermilion border need specialist management to ensure optimal and aesthetic healing.

Where pieces of tooth are missing, then gentle palpation of the soft tissues will help identify if they are lodged in the lip, cheek, or tongue. Further diagnosis will require the use of dental radiographs of the teeth and/or soft tissues of the lip. If there is concern that the tooth or a tooth fragment has been inhaled, a chest x-ray may be required.

3.9   Management of Trauma to the Primary Teeth

Primary teeth start to exfoliate from approximately the age of six, with the anterior teeth exfoliating first. Therefore, it is unlikely they are going to present a significant problem with regard to sport-related dental trauma. However, it is worth reviewing the management principles.

3.9.1   Dental Hard Tissue Injuries of Primary Teeth

Simple fractures of the tooth can be managed by either smoothing off any sharp edges, or covering over the exposed dentine. More significant injuries causing loss of pulp vitality are usually managed by extraction of the tooth. Pulp treatment in an anterior primary tooth can be difficult to carry out in a young child and the evidence for success is lacking. It also carries the risk of damage to the developing permanent tooth.

3.9.2   Periodontal Ligament Injuries

Very loose primary teeth are usually extracted, avulsed primary teeth are not usually replanted. Splinting teeth in this age group can be difficult and is difficult to justify if natural exfoliation of the tooth is imminent. Intruded teeth are usually left to re-erupt, which happens in most cases. If they do not re-erupt after several months then they are usually removed. Where teeth are displaced laterally, but still in the socket, they may be left if the displacement is not severe, or removed if the tooth is interfering with the bite and eating.

Any injury to a primary tooth carries with it the risk of damage to the underlying permanent tooth if the primary tooth root is forced into the developing permanent tooth germ. The risk of damage to the permanent tooth reduces the older a child becomes, as the permanent tooth gets closer to final development. Therefore, it is unlikely in this group when considering sport-related dental trauma. However, it is not impossible. Adverse outcomes can include damage to the crown of the underlying tooth, derangement of the position of the underlying tooth or distortion and/or shortening of the root.

Dental management in this group can be particularly challenging because of the younger age range. Some children are able to tolerate dental care whilst awake, just using dental injections. However some will not and further management may require the use of sedation or general anaesthetic.

3.10   Dental Management of Trauma to the Permanent Teeth

As previously stated, injuries can be divided into hard tissue dental injuries or periodontal ligament injuries. Both may occur at the same time, but it is useful to consider them separately because of the differences in pathology, management, and prognosis.

3.10.1 Hard Tissue Injuries

These can be classified as crown fractures into enamel, dentine, pulp, or root fractures.

3.10.1.1 Principles of Management of Crown Fractures

The underlying aim of treatment of any crown fracture (Figure 3.3) is to maintain pulp health and then to restore the aesthetics and function of the tooth. If the pulp becomes necrotic then the tooth will need a root filling or possibly even extraction. Root-filled teeth are weaker than teeth with healthy pulps. Furthermore, if the pulp loses vitality before the root has completed growth then the tooth will have thin root walls. This makes any subsequent root filling more complicated to carry out and increases the risk of fracture or other problems.

The tooth may lose pulp vitality either as a result of the initial traumatic impact damaging the blood supply to the pulp or because the pulp becomes exposed to bacterial contamination as a result of the injury. Bacteria can obviously gain access to the pulp if it is visible following an injury. However, they can also track down the tubules in the dentine if this is exposed. These injuries may not seem as severe, but sealing exposed dentine is as important as sealing an exposed pulp. Speed is of the essence. Exposed dentine or pulp that is disinfected and sealed shortly after the trauma by a dentist in the appropriate setting is likely to have much better outcomes than those teeth where treatment is delayed for more than a day.

3.10.1.2 Principles of Management of Root Fractures

Root fractures (Figure 3.4) present a different set of problems. Here the pulp is not exposed to bacterial contamination, but may still lose vitality if the injury disrupts the blood supply to the pulp. The emphasis in root fracture management is on ensuring the fractured portion is in the correct position and then stabilising it by splinting the affected tooth in an attempt to achieve healing.

3.10.2 Hard Tissue Injuries: Emergency and Long-term Management

3.10.2.1 Crown Fractures just into Enamel

Minor fractures that do not involve the pulp or the dentine will need cosmetic replacement of the fractured piece or smoothing /

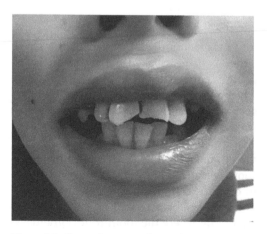

Figure 3.3 Crown fractures of central incisors.

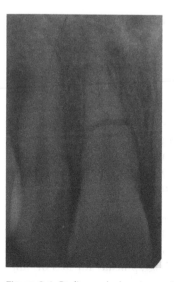

Figure 3.4 Radiograph showing root fracture in the middle part of a tooth.

polishing. Patients may well be symptom-free. Occasionally the tooth can appear to be cracked (an infraction), but otherwise whole. These teeth should still be checked by a dentist as the tooth will still have received a significant blow.

- *Emergency management:* Seek dental help when convenient
- *Dental management:* Repair or polish the tooth. Review clinically and radiographically for loss of pulp vitality.

3.10.2.2 Crown Fractures with Dentine Involvement

More significant fracture with the underlying dentine exposed (yellowish in colour when compared to the white enamel). Likely to be sensitive to hot and cold.

- *Emergency management:* Seek dental help the same day.
- *Dental management:* Seal the exposed dentine using a dental composite material. If the pulp is visible through the dentine (pinkish in colour) consider placing a calcium hydroxide lining. Rebuild the crown with a composite to prevent the adjacent tooth tipping into the space and improve aesthetics. Review clinically and radiographically for loss of pulp vitality.

3.10.2.3 Crown Fractures with Pulp Involvement

Significant injury with exposed pulp tissue. Likely to be acutely sensitive to hot, cold and touch.

- *Emergency management:* Seek dental help as soon as possible.
- *Dental management:* Cover the exposed pulp with a calcium hydroxide material to aid disinfection of the pulp and promote subsequent healing. Seal this and the exposed dentine with dental composite. Rebuild the crown with a composite to prevent the adjacent tooth tipping into the space and improve aesthetics. Review clinically and radiographically for loss of pulp vitality.

3.10.2.4 Root Fractures

The fracture could be anywhere along the length of the root and may be difficult to distinguish from a tooth that is partial avulsed at the time of injury.

- *Emergency management:* If displaced, the tooth crown should ideally be pushed into the correct position and held in place by asking the patient to bite onto a rolled swab/gauze etc. This may not be possible, either because it is too uncomfortable or because the child is too anxious or upset. Seek dental help as soon as possible.
- *Dental management:* Definitive diagnosis of a root fracture will require dental radiographs. Once this is confirmed then the displaced portion of the tooth should be put back into place, this might require local anaesthetic. In most cases the fractured portion is then splinted in place by attaching the affected tooth to a tooth either side using a piece of semi-flexible wire attached to the tooth with dental composite. Splinting times vary but are usually no more than a few weeks. The exception is where the fracture happens close to the gum line. In this case the fractured portion can be splinted for up to 4 months in an attempt to get reattachment with the periodontal cuff of tissue around the tooth. All types of fracture will need regular clinical and radiographic review.

3.10.3 Periodontal Ligament Injuries

The periodontal ligament can be damaged either by being crushed, e.g. intrusion, or by being separated from its blood supply, e.g. when a tooth is completely avulsed from its socket. Once the periodontal ligament is irreparably damaged, it cannot be restored. This results in the tooth root coming into direct contact with the alveolar bone. This root then experiences resorption mediated by osteoclasts from the alveolus. This resorption can be characterised as either surface resorption where the tooth root is gradually eaten away, or replacement resorption where the tooth becomes fused to the bone (ankylosis).

Crush injuries of the periodontal ligament are difficult to manage. The periodontal ligament cells are usually damaged beyond repair, often the best we can do is mitigate any symptoms and manage the outcome. Separation-type periodontal ligament injuries (e.g. following avulsion) offer some hope, as it is possible to restore the blood supply to the periodontal ligament cells, as long as this happens before the cells on the tooth root die.

Aside from replanting the tooth in avulsion injuries, the other principal intervention in teeth with periodontal ligament injuries is the prophylactic removal of the pulp, where there is a risk it might be compromised. Teeth with periodontal ligament damage often experience a small amount of surface root resorption that can be self-limiting. If the pulp becomes infected and/or inflamed this can greatly accelerate this resorption and increase the amount of root affected.

Unlike hard tissue injuries, some periodontal ligament injuries can remain undiagnosed until the developing problem becomes critical. For example, root resorption is often symptomless as the pulp does not lose vitality; it can only be detected on radiographs. Hence follow-up investigations for this sort of injury are critical.

3.10.4 Periodontal Ligament Injuries: Emergency and Long-term Management

3.10.4.1 Mobile Tooth (Subluxation)
Loose tooth, but still in the correct position. Tender to bite on.

- *Emergency management:* Hold the tooth in place by asking the patient to bite onto a rolled swab/gauze etc. Seek dental help the same day (particularly if excessively mobile).
- *Dental management:* The tooth will need to be supported with a splint if it is excessively mobile. Otherwise it should firm up

by itself over the next few days. Radiographic follow-up by a dentist is critical to monitor changes in the periodontal ligament and root.

3.10.4.2 Horizontal or Vertically Displaced Tooth (Lateral Luxation or Extrusive Luxation)
The tooth is either pushed forward or backwards, or could appear to be extruded. It may or may not be mobile. It may not be possible for the affected individual to close their mouth properly as the displaced tooth interferes with the bite. Difficult clinically to distinguish between this and a root fracture (emergency management is the same).

- *Emergency management:* The best emergency management is to push the tooth into the correct position using finger pressure, and then hold it in place by asking the patient to bite onto a rolled swab/gauze etc. This may not be possible, either because it is too uncomfortable or because the child is too anxious or upset. Seek dental help immediately.
- *Dental management:* If still displaced or extruded it is important to get it back to the original position if at all possible. This gets more difficult and uncomfortable the longer the time that elapses from the original injury so early dental treatment is important. Repositioning the tooth is likely to need local anaesthetic. The tooth will then need to be supported with a splint for several weeks. Radiographic follow-up is critical to monitor changes in the periodontal ligament and root.

3.10.4.3 Intruded Tooth
The tooth appears pushed into the gum so that some or even all of the crown is buried. There may or may not be discomfort, but because the tooth is out of the bite it does not tend to interfere with eating.

- *Emergency management:* Seek dental help the same day.
- *Dental management:* These are difficult injuries to manage with a poor outcome.

This is principally a crush injury of the periodontal ligament, in addition the blood supply to the pulp can also be damaged leading to a loss of pulp vitality. Mild intrusions (1–2 mm) can be left and the teeth may well re-erupt over a period of weeks. If they do not re-erupt then they may need to be extruded surgically. Severe intrusions may benefit from immediate surgical extrusion. In both cases a splint may be required if the tooth is mobile or tender to touch and, as before, regular radiographic review is need. If the intrusion is severe and the likelihood of loss of pulp vitality is high, you may consider prophylactically removing the pulp of the tooth to reduce the risk of subsequent pulp death exacerbating any external resorption. Radiographic follow-up is critical to monitor changes in the periodontal ligament and root.

3.10.4.4 Avulsed Tooth

The tooth is completely displaced from the mouth.

- *Emergency management:* Ideally the tooth should be replaced as soon as possible in order to preserve the periodontal ligament cells and promote revascularisation of the pulp.
  - Pick up the tooth by the crown only.
  - If the tooth is covered in debris consider quickly rinsing with water (no more than a few seconds). Do not try and physically remove debris from the root as this might further damage the periodontal ligament.
  - Replace the tooth and get the patient to bite onto a swab to hold it in place.
  - See a dentist as soon as possible for radiographs and splinting of the affected tooth (Figure 3.5).

  Sometimes this is not possible, particularly if the child is very distressed. If this is the case then they should attend the dentist as soon as possible so that the tooth can be replaced using local anaesthetic if required. The tooth must be stored into a solution that will keep the periodontal ligament cells alive for as long as possible.

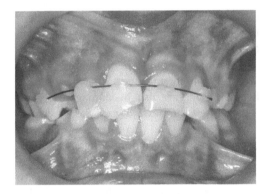

Figure 3.5 Simple wire and composite splint.

Milk, is often cited as the ideal solution as it is readily available to members of the public. Any room temperature solution that will support cell vitality will technically do. Interestingly there is some limited evidence to show that an oral rehydration solution may be effective [7]. Water should be avoided; if no other storage medium is available then the patient's saliva could be used. The patient needs to have the tooth replaced as soon as possible – 60 minutes is often quoted as the upper time limit, but it is likely that any time interval greater than 20 minutes is going to lead to an unfavourable outcome.

- *Dental management:* Irrigate the socket to remove any blood clots, then replace the tooth, if this has not already happened, and splint for 1–2 weeks. If there is a risk that the pulp may be compromised (e.g. mature root development or prolonged dry time) then the tooth should have the pulp removed. In cases where the periodontal ligament cells are almost certainly going to be dead (e.g. greater than one hour dry time) then the pulp can be removed and the root filling placed into the tooth before it is replanted as there is no time pressure anymore. Systemic antibiotics are recommended in some trauma guidelines, but the evidence for this is weak and their benefit unclear. Radiographic follow-up is critical to monitor changes in the periodontal ligament and root.

3.10.4.5 Fracture of the Alveolar Process

Mobility of several adjacent teeth is common, with perhaps an obvious change in the occlusal plane. It may not be possible for the affected individual to close their mouth properly.

- *Emergency management:* If possible push the tooth into the correct position using finger pressure, and then hold it in place by asking the patient to bite onto a rolled swab/gauze etc. This may not be possible, either because it is too uncomfortable or because the child is too anxious or upset. Seek dental help immediately.
- *Dental management:* The teeth should be correctly repositioned and then splinted; this may require local anaesthetic. As with any dental trauma, long-term clinical and radiographic follow-up is required. If managed correctly and conservatively these do not seem to be associated with significant long-term complications [8]. Because the whole alveolar process fractures, the periodontal ligament is often undamaged.

3.11 Prognosis of Trauma in Young People

Prognosis for any tooth following dental trauma will depend on the type and severity of the injury, the treatment received, and, importantly, the timing of that treatment [3]. The long-term outcomes of most traumatic dental injuries are improved if treatment is provided rapidly. Outcomes following dental trauma are many and varied and can include infection, discolouration, resorption, pulp canal obliteration, and tooth loss. Even if teeth are restored successfully, they will still require lifelong management and repair. They are also more vulnerable to further trauma and are more likely to experience problems such as crown fracture.

As a general rule of thumb, simple dental hard tissue fractures tend to cause fewer long-term problems than injuries involving the pulp. Injuries involving the pulp increase the likelihood of bacterial ingress into the tooth and loss of pulp vitality. Loss of pulp vitality ultimately weakens a tooth making it more likely to fracture. Periodontal injuries, particularly crush-type injuries, have even poorer outcomes, with teeth either experiencing resorption or ankylosis. This often results in early loss of the tooth. The only periodontal ligament injury that can have a good outcome is a separation type, i.e. avulsion, but this is dependent on effective and timely initial management.

A common question from athletes is 'when is it safe to return to sport?' There is no easy answer to this as any subsequent trauma is likely to further compromise already damaged teeth, irrespective of how recent the last trauma was. One simple indicator of fitness to return to training is whether the athlete is able to wear a mouthguard or not. If the affected tooth requires splinting for several weeks thus preventing mouthguard wear, then perhaps they should avoid the risk of further injury. However, partaking in sport is ultimately a key part of a healthy lifestyle and should therefore be encouraged, perhaps accepting the risk of further dental trauma. Clearly, any individual who has had dental trauma previously should wear a mouthguard or take other precautions as appropriate.

References

1 International Association of Dental Traumatology (IADT). (2017). Dental Trauma Guidelines.www.iadt-dentaltrauma.org/1-9%20%20IADT%20 GUIDELINES%20Combined%20-%20 LR%20-%2011-5-2013.pdf. Last accessed June 2017.
2 Al Qahtani, S. (2009). Atlas of human tooth development and eruption. atlas.dentistry. qmul.ac.uk/content/english/atlas_of_tooth_

development_in_English.pdf. Last accessed January 2017

3 Lam, R. (2016). Epidemiology and outcomes of traumatic dental injuries: a review of the literature. *Australian Dental Journal* 61: 4–20.

4 Petti, S. (2015). Over two hundred million injuries to anterior teeth attributable to large overjet: a meta-analysis. *Dental Traumatology* 31: 1–8.

5 Rahimi-Nedjat, R.K., Sagheb, K., Jacobs, C., Walter, C. (2016). Association between eruption state of the third molar and the occurrence of mandibular angle fractures. *Dental Traumatology* 32: 347–352.

6 Alnaggar, D., Andersson, L. (2015). Emergency management of traumatic dental injuries in 42 countries *Dental Traumatology* 31: 89–96

7 Jabarifar, S.E., Razavi, S.M., Haje Norouzali Tehrani, M., Roayaei Ardekani, M. (2015). The effect of oral rehydration solution on apoptosis of periodontal ligament cells. *Dental Traumatology* 31: 283–287.

8 Lauridsen, E., Gerds, T., Ove Andreasen, J. (2016). Alveolar process fractures in the permanent dentition. Part 2. The risk of healing complications in teeth involved in an alveolar process fracture. *Dental Traumatology* 32: 128–139.

4

Restoration of Teeth Damaged by Trauma
Robert Stone

4.1   Introduction

The restoration of a tooth or teeth damaged by trauma can be challenging. However, I believe if we adhere to certain basic principles the rationale for a preferred approach becomes clearer.

The first principle is conservation and by that I mean conservation of the vitality of the tooth, as well as conservation of tooth structure; both aspects are clearly inter-related [1]. For too long restorative dentistry has been concerned with the removal of healthy tooth structure to achieve functional and aesthetic outcomes. Traditional approaches were led by a desire to optimise the physical properties of restorative materials rather than optimising the strength of the underlying tooth structure. GV Black's six rules for cavity preparation were designed to optimise the restorative material, in this case amalgam, not the tooth, which often suffered immeasurably [1].

The second principle is to use a 'biomimetic' approach [2]. In this approach the restorative dentist attempts to recover the original physical, functional and aesthetic properties of the tooth. This is achieved by using the materials that best mimic the naturally occurring substrates of dentine and enamel, and draw them into a union that replicates that which we see occurring in nature. This is not a new concept and has been practiced all over the world since time immemorial. However, in dental terms this practice has been greatly aided by the advent of adhesive bonding techniques. A modern approach should allow us to augment teeth so that they are restored to their natural glory.

The third principle is to work from final form. The use of a diagnostic wax-up to determine the final form allows us to visualise shape, the key determinant in aesthetics, and assess function. Additionally it allows us to observe and control tooth reduction so that the correct amount is removed to allow for the desired restorative material. Lastly, final form allows us to break down and control the restoration of a tooth with greater certainty of outcome and the ability to retrace our steps, should we deviate.

The fourth principle is to consider how the restoration is going to fail before embarking on the restoration. On considering this aspect, one would prefer the least damaging mode of failure. A material failure that can be repaired or a portion that could be rebonded is preferable to a root that has fractured vertically or dentine substrate that has been softened by secondary caries.

Undoubtedly, the greatest step forward in the restoration of traumatised anterior teeth was the advent of dental bonding. Dr Michael Buonocore first introduced the acid etch technique in 1955 [3]. At the time he was said to have imagined a future where a dentist could 'treat a fractured anterior tooth using a

Sports Dentistry: Principles and Practice, First Edition. Edited by Peter D. Fine, Chris Louca and Albert Leung.
© 2019 John Wiley & Sons Ltd. Published 2019 by John Wiley & Sons Ltd.
Companion website: www.wiley.com/go/fine/sports_dentistry

material with which we, like an artist with a brush, could build-up that tooth to its natural form rather than (using) a pin or large crown' [4]. In his paper he described acid etching the enamel for 30 seconds using 85% phosphoric acid to produce selective dissolution of the hydroxyapatite enamel prisms, and provide a micromechanically rough surface for bonding. Over the years this process has changed very little, albeit we now use 37% phosphoric acid. The profession has grown to trust enamel bonding.

Concurrently, efforts to bond to dentine have proved more problematic. Early resins adhered cohesively to the smear layer with bond strengths in the region of 5–10 MPa. However, the polymerisation stresses of light-cured composite resins were in the region of 15–17 MPa; this often resulted in de-bonding, post-operative sensitivity, marginal staining and secondary caries [4].

The first attempts to etch the dentine produced disappointing results with bond strengths in the region of 5–10 MPa again. Although the etching removed the smear layer to expose the dentinal tubules, the etching process also transformed the hard mineralised surface into a soft mess of collagen fibrils that were inherently difficult to bond to, particularly if dried. There was little progress until the 1980s when Nakabayashi et al. [5] described the 'hybrid layer'. This layer consisted of demineralised dentine containing collagen fibrils that had been infiltrated with resin. The technique involved water rinsing and not over-drying, to maintain a collagenous matrix that when cured and stabilised, ultimately contained resin tags and collagen fibrils, in a mixture or hybrid layer.

At the same time in Japan Fusayama [6] suggested etching the enamel and dentine at the same time. He called this the total etch technique. However, the requirement to dry the enamel leads to collapse of the collagenous matrix. This he solved by applying priming agents to expand and give volume to the matrix.

At this point, dentine bonding became a three-stage process: total etch and rinse, prime and evaporate, then apply a resin bonding agent before light curing to stabilise. By the early 1990s, studies by Kanka et al. suggested that wet bonding improved the bond strengths significantly, but it was still a very difficult balancing act to judge what was too wet, too dry, or just right [7,8]. Further developments were often practical and time-saving, such a combining the primer and bond in the same bottle to create a two-stage technique. Others were a modernised return to the past by attempting to partially dissolve and bond to the smear layer using self-etching primer adhesive. These systems were designed to be used on dry dentine and the gentle etching of the smear layer was thought to not remove the smear plugs and greatly reduced post-operative sensitivity. Finally came a generation of all-in-one self-etching, self-priming, self-adhesive systems. These far more acidic systems were thought to have problems with incomplete monomer conversion and were often thought to need to be too thick to polymerise completely. This could lead to increased water absorption and lower bond strengths.

All of the changes relating to the different generations of dentine bonding suggest to me that the substrate is inherently difficult to deal with and should not be too heavily relied upon. Albeit there are good arguments to attempt to allow dentine to provide the very best bonding it can, by better understanding of the substrate and utilising concepts such as immediate dentine sealing, if possible.

4.2 Principle Components of Modern Composite Resins

1) Dimethacrylate resin, usually bisphenol A glycidyl methacrylate (BisGMA) and urethane dimethacrylate (UMDA). In 1962 Bowen synthesised BisGMA. This large hydrophobic dimethacrylate monomer or its derivations, such as UMDA form the basis of modern day composite resins.
2) Filler particles were originally quartz; modern fillers are based on barium and

strontium glasses, partly because they are radiopaque. Unfortunately these metallic salts lead to the degradation of the glass. Various sizes of filler particles give the restoration adequate physical and mechanical properties.

3) Polymerisation initiators, initially chemically based around benzoyl peroxide and a tertiary amine. Nowadays, photo-initiation using a blue light (wavelength 460–470 nm) is widespread. This system depends on the excitation of a diketone, usually camphorquinone, by the light, to react with a tertiary amine to bring about polymerisation. Light activation allows for controlled setting. However, it has several pitfalls, such as premature polymerisation from operating or other external light sources, inadequate exposure to the light, and variation in the depth of the cure.

4) Coupling agents, usually a silane, that bonds the filler to the resin matrix. This is very important as it allows the transfer of stress from the resin to the filler and maintains the integrity of the material.

Other components include inhibitors, to prevent premature resin polymerisation and colour stabilizers.

4.3 Restorative Techniques

4.3.1 Reattachment of Fractured Teeth

Reattachment of the broken fragment is highly conservative, truly biomimetic, defines final form immediately, and the mode of failure has no further adverse effects (Figure 4.1).

The reattachment approach can be used for both uncomplicated (not involving the pulp) and complicated crown fractures. The ability of the original fragment to fit back together accurately and the location of the fracture (not supragingival) are the limiting features. Providing the fractured portion realigns accurately, a simple bonding procedure will restore the original aesthetics, shape, colour, surface texture, and lustre. Additionally, the psychological impact of retaining the original tooth cannot be underestimated.

Reis et al. stated that simple reattachment with no further preparation of the fragment or tooth was able to restore only 37.1% of the original tooth's fracture resistance, but a buccal chamfer recovered 60.6% of that fracture resistance, and bonding with an overlapping veneer of composite restored the tooth's fracture strength to 97.2% [9]. Clinical issues concern whether to bevel or chamfer the buccal margins, substrate preparation, substrate conditioning, and which material one should use to achieve a durable bond. My preference is to bond the fractured portions together using warmed restorative composite (a submicron hybrid). Finishing and polishing techniques will be discussed and shown later.

4.3.2 Layered Composite Build-up/Class IV

Dr Buonocores prophesy has come true. Over 50 years of innovation and technological

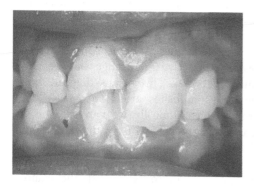
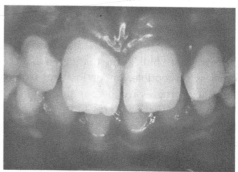

Figure 4.1 Clinical example and images of reattachment.

advances in aesthetic composite restorations mean that dentists today can build up a fractured anterior tooth using a multitude of composite materials. Different shades, opacities, translucencies, stains, and textures exist; often within one composite system. The results that can be obtained are truly remarkable and must be the first thought when considering how to restore anterior teeth damaged by trauma.

Early composites were simply one shade and the dentist had to pick the best match. Nowadays systems have the potential to deliver all the nuances of a natural tooth. Multi-layered systems can rival ceramics, but require time and training to become proficient. Some dentists argue that they are too time-consuming and unpredictable, and prefer to use indirect laboratory-based procedures that are often less conservative of tooth structure.

The layering approach first described by Lorenzo Vanini and later by Didier Dietchi provides a controlled technique to optimise the advanced composite systems now available [10,11]. These advanced systems usually comprise dentine varieties, enamel varieties, and intermediate modifying effects. The systems were first developed with dental technicians in mind, to be used indirectly, as they correlate closely to their familiar porcelain build-up systems. However, clinicians soon realised that with good isolation and careful planning these systems could lend themselves to direct work.

As previously discussed, basic principles should be followed. The conservation of tooth structure is paramount. Tooth preparation should be limited to a buccal 0.5 mm chamfer or a bevel. My preference is for a chamfer as this allows for more bulk at the margin and is therefore less susceptible, under loading, to flex and cause progressive de-bonding and discolouration, as we see with the bevel preparation. Additionally I like to polish the chamfer margin with a white stone and silicone points as I feel it improves the optical properties at the margin. On the palatal surface a smooth butt fit is adequate and should not be

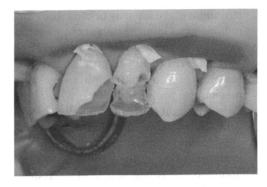

Figure 4.2 Palatal composite baskets.

chamfered unless the trauma has naturally produced an inclined plane.

Final tooth preparation can be achieved after careful isolation with a rubber dam, and my preference is to sandblast the tooth with 50 micron aluminium oxide powder.

Biomimetic principles are observed with the multi-layered systems as the different composites represent dentine and enamel. Care should be taken to recreate the anatomy as carefully as possible. However, some variations are often required. These variations are a result of the differences in the refractive index of the materials and natural teeth.

The refractive index is governed by how much a wavelength bends when passing through a material; this has an impact on the appearance of natural or restorative materials by affecting their light-scattering characteristics and translucency. For example, water has a refractive index of 1.33 and glass, 1.52. The refractive index of human enamel is 1.62. The refractive index increases as the tooth dehydrates (Figures 4.3 and 4.4). This causes the tooth to become whiter and more opaque. In studies of enamel composites, the average refractive index ranges between 1.49 and 1.541 [12]. This means that the most enamel composites are more 'glassy' and translucent. Clinically we can see this as greying in the enamel from the darkness in the mouth. To eliminate this effect I would always suggest overbuilding the dentine composite layer so as to keep the enamel layer much thinner than anatomically correct;

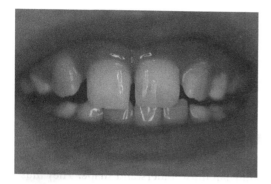

Figure 4.3 Dehydrated teeth.

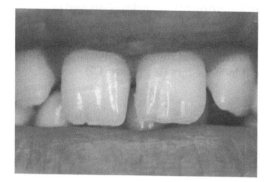

Figure 4.4 Rehydrated teeth.

roughly 50% of the anatomical thickness. However, manufacturers have identified this weakness and several brands have developed enamel composite with refractive indices more closely aligned to natural enamel, for example Micerium, developed Enamel Plus HRi (High Refractive Index). This material can be placed to much more anatomically correct thicknesses. Thus making these materials even more biomimetic.

Lastly, the concept of working from final form is crucial to allow the clinician to carefully control the composite build-up. With shapes and anatomical thickness paramount, the clinician can ill afford to have to make large adjustments to the incisal edge position, buccal contour, or palatal surface. If a diagnostic wax-up is made, a putty matrix can be produced. This approach has several distinct advantages. Firstly, it provides a surface to accurately reproduce the palatal surface of the tooth; thereby ensuring the

occlusal contacts and loading are controlled and should require very little adjustment. Secondly, the putty index allows the clinician to produce a palatal basket of enamel (Figure 4.2) that can be filled in with anatomically correct volumes of dentine composite, characterised internally and finally layered with the correct volume of enamel composite. A far cry for the days of balancing some composite on your finger, zapping it with the light, and shaping it up!

However, the production of a diagnostic wax-up takes time and this can be problematic. With a trauma case, the patient and often the parents of the patient are most keen to restore the tooth or teeth immediately. However, I find with a careful explanation, the advantages are clear. These include the need to produce a template to control the restoration build-up, the advantage in letting a little time pass so that any soft tissue injuries begin to heal, and a period of time to correctly assess the pulp vitality. My approach is as follows: at the first appointment I try to take good history, examine the patient and make the correct diagnosis. I then explain my findings, clean and cover the dentine, usually with some glass ionomer cement, and finally I take alginate impressions. From the casts I can produce a diagnostic wax-up that is both aesthetically correct, and gives me the correct occlusal relationship. This wax-up can be used to form a putty index.

Lastly, if we consider the mode of failure of Class IV composite restorations; there are few serious consequences. The potential lost time and financial consequences are obvious, although it is often possible to rebond the restored fragment if retained by the patient. According to the studies failure is a reality. The longevity of large Class IV composite restorations that have been placed on fractured anterior teeth has been shown to be relatively short. Robertson et al. evaluated 140 Class IV restorations over a 15-year period and found that all the restorations had been replaced at least once throughout the study, and some on multiple occasions [13]. In a systematic review by DeMarco et al., they looked at anterior composite studies, with follow-up ranging from 3 to 17 years and found failure rates ranged from 53.4% to 100% [14]. Spinas et al. followed-up 70 Class IV restorations placed in traumatised teeth and found they had a 100% failure rate. Sadly they concluded that 'composites cannot be used for long-term restorations; if the subject has completed his growth, the mandatory therapeutic alternatives are prosthetic restorations (crowns, porcelain veneers)' [15].

Personally, as long as the patient is aware of the downsides, a less-damaging mode of failure is vitally important. In my opinion this remains critically important, even if you do decide to progress to a different restorative modality.

4.4 Success with Anterior Composite Restorations

The key to an aesthetic Class IV build-up can be broken down into four elements: shape, shade, surface texture, and polishing.

4.4.1 Shape

To be able to artistically recreate a tooth, the clinician must understand shape. They must be able to recreate the anatomical features seen in anterior teeth, such as the labio-incisal ridge, proximal line angles, V-shaped grooves, lobes, cervical marginal ridge, twists in the labial surface, sloping marginal ridge, proximal groove and transitional line angles, different incisal edges (see Figure 4.5).

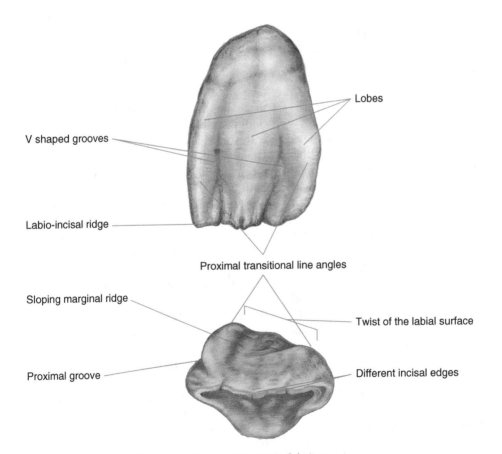

Figure 4.5 Anterior tooth anatomy. Illustrated by Jurgita Sybaite.

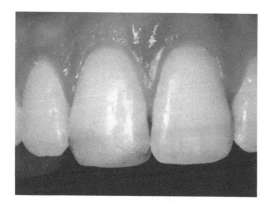

Figure 4.6 A Class IV restoration before.

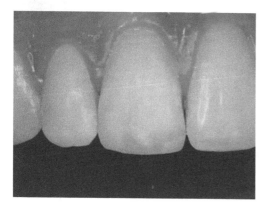

Figure 4.7 The final composite restoration.

The best way to achieve this goal is to define the final form of the restoration and tooth using a diagnostic wax-up. A diagnostic wax-up has several advantages, but in particular that the palatal form and occlusal contacts can be formed in wax and translated using a putty index to the mouth.

4.4.2 Shade

The colour of a tooth is a complex and multi-faceted interaction between the incident light waves that are reflected, scattered, and refracted. This will be subtly different in natural dentine and enamel as well as the different restorative enamels, dentines, and bonding resins (Figures 4.6 and 4.7).

A good understanding of the human eye is relevant to which of these facets should take

priority. The human eye is sensitive to visible light, wavelengths between 380 and 770 nm on the electromagnetic spectrum, the light photons are refracted by the lens and are focused on the retina. On the retina the light is interpreted by 125 million black-and-white sensitive cells known as rods in addition to six million colour sensitive cells known as cones. This means that the black/white-sensitive rods outnumber the colour-sensitive cones by 20:1. The name given to the black-and-white scale is the value; so value is how dark and how light an object is. The name given to the actual colour is the hue and the intensity of the hue is known as the chroma. With this information we can understand why the human eye is much more sensitive to subtle variations in the value of a tooth rather than minor differences in the hue and chroma.

So when assessing the shade of a tooth the first thing, and most important aspect, to assess is the value. A useful verification trick is to place a small amount of the dentine and enamel composite you have chosen on the tooth that you are trying to mimic. Then take an image and convert it to black and white; this will allow you to assess if the composite you have selected is the correct value.

Hue is the name of the colour. This corresponds to the wavelength of light reflected by the teeth and detected by the observer. Early multi-layer composite systems had different dentine hues. However, Yamamoto, and later Touati et al., both observed that over 80% of natural teeth corresponded most closely to the orange-yellow hue of a Vita A shade [16,17]. Nowadays all the systems have moved to offering one universal dentine hue, but with a range of chroma. In this day of bleached white teeth, the hue is becoming less important as it is very difficult to interpret hue at very low (white) intensity.

Chroma describes the saturation of hue. Chroma and value are inversely related; as the intensity of chroma increases, the value decreases (becomes darker). The chroma of a natural tooth principally comes from the dentine; this then altered by the thickness and opacity of the overlying enamel. Where the enamel is thin, at the gingival third, the chroma is greatest. Incisally, where the enamel is thickest the chroma is most diminished. This creates a chroma gradient within the tooth. Increasing opacity of the enamel, as seen with dehydration and bleaching, can exaggerate the chroma gradient. Thinning of the enamel with age increases the translucency and increases the dominance of the chroma from the dentine.

The dentine also influences the opacity of the tooth and is important to mimic in the restorative material. Incident light travels through the more translucent enamel and is reflected by the more opaque dentine. This can often be seen as lobes or comb like structures within the tooth. Some systems rely on opaque dentine shades to prevent light transmission others rely on shear bulk of dentine to prevent the darkness of the mouth greying out the restored tooth.

The enamel influences the chroma and value, but is also critical to the translucency of the tooth or restoration. The translucency of enamel is principally influenced by the thickness. Within an individual tooth this can range from 0.2 mm in the cervical third and up to 1.5 mm in the incisal third.

However, over the lifetime of the tooth the enamel thins and consequently becomes more translucent. This translucency decreases values by increasing the influence of dentine chroma and appearing dark owing to the lack of light emanating from the mouth. Therefore enamel is the dominant modifying factor over time. Young teeth are lighter, whiter and less translucent, and older teeth are darker, more chromatic and more translucent. Adult teeth lie somewhere in a very varied spectrum in between.

Opalescence is type of dichroism seen when short wavelength light is reflected and scattered in highly translucent material. Transmitted light appears as yellowish-red and scattered light appears blue (see Figures 4.8 and 4.9).

Hydroxyapatite crystals provided the highly translucent material for this effect to occur in. While the phenomenon will occur

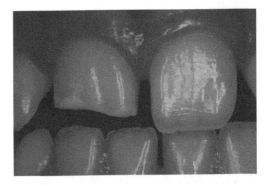

Figure 4.8 Opalescence in natural teeth.

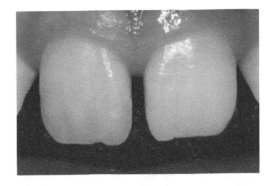

Figure 4.9 An attempt to recreate the effect in composite.

throughout the enamel, it is most frequently observed in the incisal third where the dentine has no influence.

Another feature seen in teeth and desirable in a restoration is *fluorescence*. The enamel and particularly the amelo-dentinal junction play an import role the transmission of light. The highly mineralised pre-dentine layer is thought to help create fluorescence when it reflects short-wavelength (ultraviolet) invisible light as slightly longer-wavelength blueish light. Some composite systems advocate the incorporation of a resin layer to help achieve this effect.

Other effects can be described as characterisation. These include lines, patches, clouds, and bands. They can be white opacities or varying translucency or a variety of colours ranging from subtle bands or dark brown cracks or fissures.

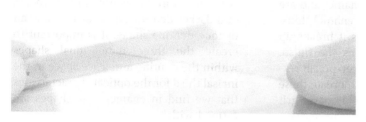

Figure 4.10 Wedges of dentine and enamel composite made from the actual material.

Successful shade taking:

1) The shade should be taken well before any treatment commences to avoid any dehydration of the teeth.
2) Ideally the light should be northern mid-day light (5500 K). This can be achieved using a variety of colour-corrected light sources.
3) Assess value first; this should be done quickly using the enamel shades against the incisal third. Squinting will help your rods dominate.
4) Chroma should also be assessed quickly, at the cervical third using the dentine shade guide, with fresh eyes that have been sensitized by looking at a complementary colour such as pale blue. Blue will help sensitize the eyes to the red-yellow-orange wavelengths.
5) A polarised filter can be helpful to assess the chroma, as this will prevent reflection and shine and allow you to assess the relative thickness of enamel.
6) Ideally use a composite system that uses shade guides that have been made from the composite material you are intending to use (Figure 4.10). It is also useful if they vary in thickness, as this will help you formulate the chroma gradient.
7) Make a note of the lustre/polish of the enamel surface.
8) Make a note of any other characteristics; this is best conveyed by taking an image of the teeth and drawing a detailed colour map.

4.4.3 Surface Texture

The surface texture of the restoration is vital in recreating a life-like effect. The shape of the tooth is principally seen by the incident light being reflected by the primary anatomical features, described above, such as the transitional line angles and the cervical bulge. These features form the face of the tooth. The other areas of the tooth deflect the light and are less obvious when viewed in three dimensions. An understanding of these primary anatomical features can also allow the clinician to create visual illusions. Reproducing symmetry and shape of the transitional areas can fool the eyes into believing teeth of different widths are the same size and shape. I like to use scalpel blades and fine grit pointed flame-shaped diamond burs. These should be used with great care to preserve the contours of the primary anatomy. I find pencil marks on the adjacent teeth help me copy the symmetry and curves while pencil marks on the restoration prevent me from removing the primary (reflective) contours and help me work into the curved deflective surfaces.

The secondary surface texture, also referred to as macrotexture, consists of the developmental lobes, their corresponding mamelons, and various developmental grooves. To achieve these features I like to use green and white stones.

Lastly, there is micro-texture. This consists of pitting and striations known as perikymata, accessory ridges, and grooves such as the imbrication lines that interrupt the cervical bulge. Once again most of these micro-texture features are confined to the enamel and are therefore lost with age as the enamel thins. Micro-texture is important, as it breaks up the reflective light and softens the finish. Care should be taken not to over-polish restorations. I find the best way to create these features is by using a hand-held coarse grit diamond burr and scratching the surface. Others recommend scoring the surface with the tip of a scalpel blade.

4.4.4 Polishing

Prior to polishing I like to ensure that the composite material is fully cured at the surface. When composite resins are cured in the presence of oxygen there is always a fine air-inhibited layer left on the surface where the composite fails to fully polymerise. This can be eliminated by curing the composite under glycerine or an aqueous jelly to block out the oxygen and render the surface fully polymerised, hard, and highly polishable.

The objective of the polishing is to create highly reflective surfaces on the correct areas of the tooth. These are the transitional line angles and other high points that serve to accentuate the macro-texture features. Care should be taken not to polish out any features, particularly the more delicate micro-textures. My polishing regime involves using a 3 micron polishing paste, followed by a 1 micron polishing paste, both applied, lightly, using a goat's-hair brush at 7000 rpm under water spray. Finally I polish the highly reflective surfaces with an aluminium oxide paste that is applied on a felt wheel with a very light touch at 8000 rpm.

4.5 Clinical Sequence

1) Form the palatal composite wall in enamel. This should be 0.2-0.3 mm thick.
2) Form the proximal surfaces in enamel to create a basket.
3) Begin to fill in the dentine in increments of a darker dentine shade or by using an opaque dentine shade. It is important to create the three dimensional shapes within the dentine and leave space in the incisal third for the optical characteristics that we find in enamel. The shapes are formed with metal instruments, silicone tips and brushes.
4) Special characterisation features are added to produce opacities, bands, cracks, fluorescence and translucencies prior to the final enamel layer. The characterisations are normally applied using very subtle volumes of flowable composites. They tend to be tints to produce stains and milky opacities or clear enamel resins to produce blue/grey transparencies.
5) The final enamel is added later. This is best added in a larger volume and compressed, to avoid incorporating air bubbles, as the volume is reduced to the correct dimension. Very slight overbuilding will allow for minor adjustments at the finishing stage.
6) Finishing, refining and enhancing the primary anatomical shape and surface texture.
7) Apply aqueous gel to air block and final cure for 60 seconds from all angles.
8) Polishing with 3 micron, 1 micron polishing pastes and the final shine added with aluminium oxide paste.

At the end of the procedure it is important to remember that the isolated tooth will have dehydrated significantly. This will make the natural teeth look very white and opaque and your new restoration darker and more translucent.

At this stage hold your nerve and trust your colour mapping and shade taking.

Often a good guide is to look at the appearance of the fully hydrated teeth in the opposing arch that have not been isolated.

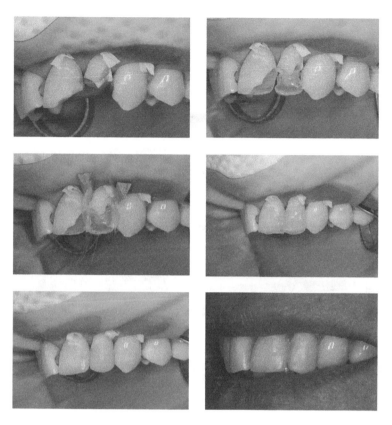

The example on the next page shows the restoration of a 12 year old boy's upper left central incisor following a fall from his bicycle.

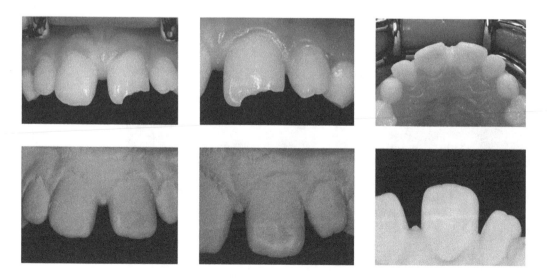

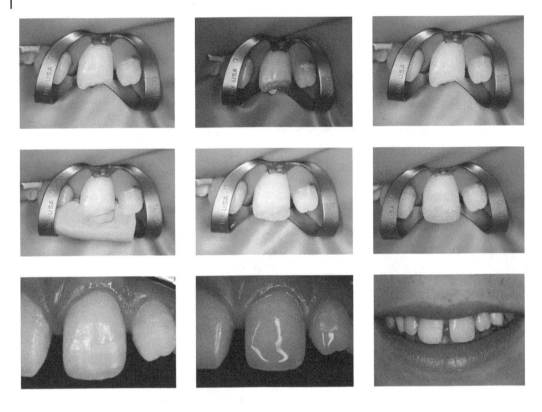

The following page shows the restoration of both the central incisors of a 46 year old lady who injured the teeth playing netball.

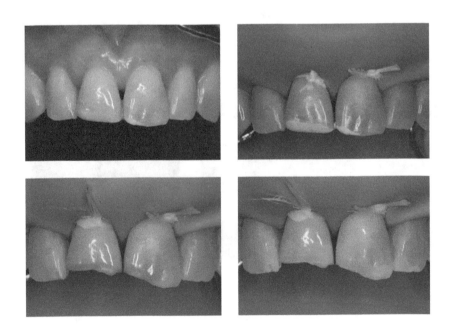

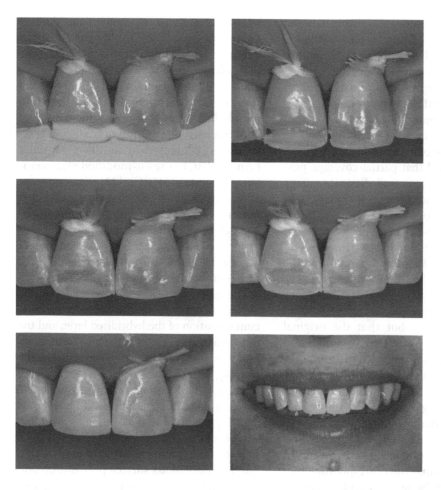

4.6 Partial Bonded Porcelain Restorations/Minimally Invasive Bonded Porcelain

If one wishes to consider indirect restorations for the reasons of long-term survival mentioned above, and alongside the potential for more enduring aesthetics, I believe there is room for minimally invasive bonded porcelain, as conceived by Sverker Toreskog some 18 years prior to his first publication in English in 2002 [18] and to some extent popularised and promoted by the Magne brothers. In his approach, Toreskog resolutely maintains the four principles of conservative dentistry.

Tooth preparation is very minimal and every attempt is made to preserve enamel. Margins are placed very supragingival to avoid exposing dentine in the cervical areas where the enamel is thinnest. Marginal preparations are as thin as 0.2 mm and a truly biomimetic replacement of enamel occurs to rebuild the tooth. Enamel bonding is trusted and dentine bonding carried out to the best of one's ability. Bonding is carried out under rubber dam isolation to optimise results. The concept relies on final-form diagnostic wax-ups to control and measure minimal tooth preparation.

This approach is very similar to the biomimetic dentistry illustrated by Pascal Magne in the late 1990s, when he described dental biomimetics as: 'the interrelationship between biology, mechanics, function and aesthetics' [19]. He explained how full crowns remove large volumes of tooth structure and provide stiff and unyielding restorations that if traumatised would lead to inevitable pulpal consequences or root injury. This was evident from the work of Alastair Stoke and John Hood on impact resistance of intact and crowned teeth [20]. He proposed that partial-coverage porcelain restoration may well dissipate energy during impact and protect the underlying tooth substrate from further damage, rather like the crumple zone in a modern car.

His early studies looked at the effect of aging, disease, and tooth preparation on the stiffness or flexibility of anterior teeth [21], and showed that the mechanical stiffness of a tooth reduces with increasing volume of buccal enamel loss, but that the original stiffness could be recovered by bonding a feldspathic porcelain veneer to the tooth.

Comparisons are made between the physical properties of the dental hard tissues and corresponding biomaterials. Magne suggested that feldspathic porcelain has physical properties most like enamel and hybrid composites have physical properties most like dentine and that the corresponding biomaterials should be used to replace natural tooth structure, with all the materials and substrates brought into one union using bonding systems.

He was circumspect about dentine bonding, but described a new method of immediate dentine sealing to maximise the bond achievable. The method involves etching, washing without over-drying, priming, and bonding using Optibond FL to produce a hybridised layer in the dentine and then allowing the hybridised layer to mature over a number of weeks. His studies showed that the in-vitro bond strengths achievable continue increasing up to seven weeks after hybridisation [19]. Final bonding of the porcelain restoration can then be carried out to optimise the enamel, by etching for 30 seconds, washing, and drying thoroughly before applying bond and curing.

The advantages of immediate dentine sealing are as follows: freshly cut and clean dentine is ideal for optimal hybridization; pre-polymerisation increases bond strengths; and a delayed placement of the final restoration allows the strength of the bond to mature in a stress-free environment. Studies show increased retention of traditional restorations cemented with glass ionomer cement (GIC) or resin-modified glass ionomer cement (RMGIC) [22]. The concept allows a clinician to concentrate on wet bonding for dentine and dry bonding for enamel. Finally, the original reason the idea as conceived by Pashley, was to protect against bacterial micro-leakage and therefore reduce post-prep sensitivity [23].

The potential disadvantages concern the ability to reattach to the hybridized layer, contamination of the hybridised layer, and the potential to affect the fit of the final restoration. However, most of these issues can be overcome by using a sandblaster to clean and refresh the hybridised layer, using a more hydrophobic bonding agent, such as Optibond FL and only applying the bond to the dentine to hybridise, while keeping the margins in enamel.

To ensure a high-quality and long-lasting bond, a meticulous surface preparation and luting procedure is required. I like to try in the ceramic restorations to assess the shape and shade. If I am happy to proceed I seek the patient's approval to progress. If they agree, I isolate the teeth and begin the substrate conditioning procedure. The porcelain is etched with 10% hydrofluoric acid for 90 seconds if it is feldspathic porcelain and only 20 seconds for lithium disilicate Emax Press. I then wash the restoration and place it in distilled water for four minutes in an ultrasonic bath. After four minutes I dry the restoration and confirm the absence of any porcelain residue from the HF etching process. If any residue is seen, I remove it by scrubbing with phosphoric acid etch for 10 seconds. I wash again and confirm a clean smooth internal fit surface.

At this point I apply a layer of silane coupling agent. I wait for this to dry naturally and apply another layer. When the silane is nearly dry I sandblast the tooth to clean and reactivate the hybridised layer. The tooth is then thoroughly washed and dried before etching with 37% phosphoric acid for 30 seconds.

The tooth is thoroughly washed again and dried for an extended period. Then I apply a layer of Optibond to the tooth and the internal fit surface of the restoration. My assistant suctions away any excess and I load the restoration with warmed (55 °C) normal light-cured composite material. I choose a shade that corresponds to the underlying dentine shade. The bonded porcelain restoration is then puddled into place and any excess gently removed. When the restoration is fully seated I cure the composite through the porcelain for an extended period (90 seconds). I tidy up the margins and remove any excess bond using a scalpel blade. Lastly I apply aqueous jelly and cure the margins in an air- inhibited environment. If there are multiple restorations, I move through this process of individual cementation one at a time.

I use normal light-cured restorative composite because it offers several advantages. Firstly, it handles very well as it cools, secondly it offers superior mechanical properties, owing to higher filler content, and lastly light-cured composite is more colour-stable than chemically cured alternatives.

A minimally invasive approach, as outlined above is the only viable alternative to direct composite restorations when restoring traumatised anterior teeth.

I believe success is dependant on working from final form to correctly assess and truly conserve tooth structure. Enamel bonding should be prioritised at all times and dentine bonding should be the best it can be by utilising immediate dentine sealing. The restorations should be cemented in a perfectly isolated environment; under rubber dam. The clinician should use a meticulous cementation protocol to gain the very best bond using normal light-cured composite. If all these steps are followed, the result should be beautiful, adequately strong, and biologically fully integrated restorations.

References

1 Black, G.V. (1908). *A Work on Operative Dentistry*. Medico Dental Publishing, Chicago.

2 Magne, P., Belser U. (2002). *Bonded Porcelain Restorations in the Anterior Dentition: A Biomimetic Approach*. Quintessssence Publishing Co., Inc., Berlin.

3 Buonocore, M. (1955). A simple method of increasing the adhesion of acrylic filling materials to enamel surfaces. *Journal of Dental Research* 34(6): 849–853.

4 Davidson, C.L., deGee, A.J., Feilzer, A.J. (1984). The competition between composite dentin bond strength and the polymerization contraction stress. *Journal of Dental Research* 63: 1396–1399.

5 Nakabayashi, N., Pashley, D.H. (1998). *Hybridization of Dental Hard Tissues*. Quintessence Publishing Co., Inc., Chicago.

6 Fusuyama, T. (1980). *New Concepts in Operative Dentistry*. Quintessence Publishing Co., Inc., Chicago.

7 Kanca, J. (1996). Wet bonding: effect of drying time and distance. *American Journal of Dentistry* 9: 273–276.

8 Kanca, J. (1996). Improved bond strength through acid etching of dentin and bonding to wet dentin surfaces. *Journal of the American Dental Association* 123: 35–43.

9 Reis, A., Loguercio, A.D., Kraul, A., Matson, E. (2004). Reattachment of fractured teeth: a review of literature regarding technique and materials. *Operative Dentistry* 29(2): 226–233.

10 Vanini, L., DeSimone, F., Tammaro, S. (1997). Indirect composite restorations in the anterior region: a predictable technique for complex cases. *Practical Periodontics and Aesthetic Dentistry* 9 (7): 795–802.

11 Dietschi, D. (2001). Layering concepts in anterior composite restorations. *Journal of Adhesive Dentistry* 3: 71–80.

12 Meng, Z., Tao, X.S., Yao, H., et al. (2009). Measurement of the refractive index of human teeth by optical coherence tomography. *Journal of Biomedical Optics* 14(3): 034010.

13 Robertson, A., Robertson, S., Norén, J.G. (1997). A retrospective evaluation of traumatized permanent teeth. *International Journal of Paediatric Dentistry* 7: 217–226.

14 Demarco, F.F., Collares, K., Coelho-de-Souza, F.H., et al. (2015). Anterior composite restorations: a systematic review on long-term survival and reasons for failure. *Dental Materials* 31(10): 1214–1224.

15 Spinas, E. (2004). Longevity of composite restorations of traumatically injured teeth. *American Journal of Dentistry* 17(6): 407–411.

16 Yamamoto, M. (1992). The value conversion system and a new concept for expressing the shades of natural teeth. *Quintessence of Dental Technology* 19(1): 2–9.

17 Touati, B., Miara, P., Nathansen, D. (1993). *Esthetic Dentistry and Ceramic Restorations*. Martin Dunitz Ltd, London, UK.

18 Toreskog, S. (2002). The minimally invasive and aesthetic bonded porcelain technique. *International Dental Journal* 52: 353–363.

19 Magne, P., So, W.S., Cascione, D. (2007). Immediate dentin sealing supports delayed restoration placement. *Journal of Prosthetic Dentistry* 98: 166–174.

20 Stokes, A.N., Hood, J.A. (1993). Impact fracture characteristics of intact and crowned human central incisors. *Journal of Oral Rehabilitation* 20: 89–95.

21 Magne, P., Douglas, W.H. (1999). Porcelain veneers: dentin bonding optimization and biomimetic recovery of the crown. *International Journal of Prosthodontics* 12(2): 111–121.

22 Magne, P. (2005). Immediate dentin sealing: a fundamental procedure for indirect bonded restorations. *Journal of Esthetic Restorative Dentistry* 17: 144–154.

23 Pashley, E.L., Comer, R.W., Simpson, M.D., et al. (1992). Dentin permeability: sealing the dentin in crown preparations. *Operative Dentistry* 17(1): 13–20.

5

Dealing with Endodontic Problems Following Sporting Trauma
Geoffrey St. George

5.1 Introduction

Damage to the teeth and jaws while participating in sport is relatively uncommon, though the chance of it happening increases in contact sports. Certain sports are designated high risk despite mouth guards being worn, e.g. rugby, martial arts and hockey, while additional protection from face masks and head guards, e.g. American football, can reduce injuries dramatically.

Teeth have two regions where trauma can cause irreparable damage: the dental pulp and periodontium. The dental pulp, contained within the root canal system of a tooth (Figure 5.1), has a number of functions:

1) *Formative*: cells in the pulp produce dentine, which forms the majority of hard tissues of the tooth.
2) *Nutrition*: the pulp contains blood vessels, which supply the living part of the tooth with nutrients.
3) *Protective*: cells within the pulp produce dentine when injury occurs.
4) *Sensory*: extremes of temperature, bacteria or trauma are detected by the nerves within the pulp and perceived as pain.

Damage to the pulp therefore stops all of these functions. This can cause teeth to stop developing, resulting in thin root walls, which may eventually fracture and cause the loss of the tooth. It also allows bacteria from the mouth to invade the root canal system, causing infection that can result in pain and swelling. When dental trauma does occur, injuries to the dental pulps of teeth are relatively common [1].

The periodontium consists of the gingiva, periodontal ligament, cementum, and alveolar bone proper (Figure 5.2). It has some functions similar to the dental pulp (formative, sensory, nutrition) but its main functions are to attach teeth to the jaws, as well as to act as a shock absorber during normal function. Damage to these tissues can cause severe complications (see later), which can be influenced by the health of the pulp. Therefore, the dentist has an important role in both preventing pulp necrosis and treating infected, necrotic pulps. The injured athletes, their sports coaches, and medical staff also have a part to play by ensuring prompt attendance at the dentist's surgery following trauma, to minimise the chances of complications, which could cause the loss of teeth.

5.2 Guidelines for Sports Doctors, Coaches, and Team Members

Ensure all team members are registered with a dentist, as hunting for a new dentist when an injury occurs can be difficult. Well maintained mouths have less gum disease and

Sports Dentistry: Principles and Practice, First Edition. Edited by Peter D. Fine, Chris Louca and Albert Leung.
© 2019 John Wiley & Sons Ltd. Published 2019 by John Wiley & Sons Ltd.
Companion website: www.wiley.com/go/fine/sports_dentistry

fillings, which can influence healing following injury.

Ensure that injuries are attended to promptly, as a delay in treatment can result in dental infections and even loss of teeth. This results in lost time from training and participation in sports.

Broken teeth, especially where their root canals have been exposed, must be attended to quickly regardless of whether they are painful or not.

Displaced teeth must be repositioned quickly, otherwise they may be impossible to move.

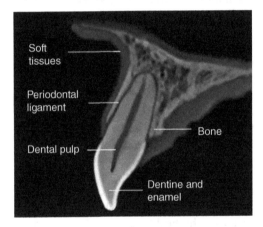

Figure 5.1 Cross-section of a tooth and supporting tissues.

Teeth knocked out of the mouth must be placed back in their sockets immediately. If they can't then they must be placed in a suitable storage medium, and the patient and tooth transported to their dentist as soon as possible.

Ensure team members attend their appointments and are followed up for review.

5.3 Nature of Injuries

The injury to a tooth and its pulp following trauma depends on:

- The direction of the trauma
- The energy of the trauma
- The size and resilience of the striking object
- Local anatomy and stage of development
- Protection from a protective mouth guard or head guard
- The restorative status of the tooth.

The contribution of each of these factors will result in damage to the tooth and its supporting tissues, which may be unique. The classification of the injury type, and signs and symptoms may not fully indicate the true extent of the injury, which may be multi-factorial.

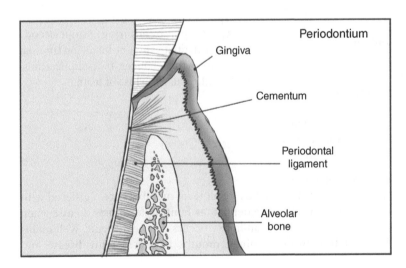

Figure 5.2 The periodontium, showing its constituent parts. *(Images courtesy of Eleanor Robson).*

Damage to a tooth is often depicted as in Figure 5.3. A horizontal blow to the tooth causes movement of the tooth about a point within the root. This results in compression or stretching/tearing of the periodontal attachment, depending on its location around the root. Compression of the periodontal ligament, cementum, and alveolar bone will cause cell death, which results in these tissues eventually being replaced, often by different cells. This leads to repair if the damage is extensive, i.e. the periodontal ligament/cementum are replaced by other cells such as those from bone or connective tissue resulting in different forms of resorption [2,3]. Alternatively, regeneration, which is where the necrotic cells are replaced with identical cells, can occur if conditions are favourable, i.e. damage is relatively limited and the correct cells required for regeneration are present locally. The nerves and blood vessels (neurovascular bundle) entering the apical foramen of the tooth can also sustain similar crushing or stretching/tearing injuries.

Most trauma to teeth is often due to a horizontal blow, which may also have a downward or upward component. The greater the upward component, the more likely the tooth is partly or fully intruded, which results in a greater amount of cells covering the tooth or structures entering the apical foramen being irreparably damaged.

In reality, due to the variability in anatomy around teeth, the degree of injury may differ considerably. Figure 5.4 shows a cone beam CT scan (CBCT) of a tooth. There is little bone on one side of the tooth, therefore the damage seen in Figure 5.3 doesn't occur. This means that the energy transferred to the tooth, rather than compressing or tearing tissues, may result in its movement or even loss of the tooth from its socket. Compare this to Figure 5.3, where a similar blow may result in the damage to the supporting tissues, or if high enough, the fracture of the tooth, root, or overlying bone.

With dental trauma, the current system, based on Andreasen's modification of the WHO classification, categorises injuries based on the tissues damaged: dental hard

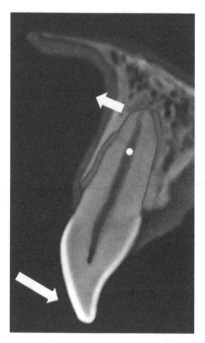

Figure 5.3 A traumatized tooth showing its rotation and areas of compression (blue), and stretching and tearing (red).

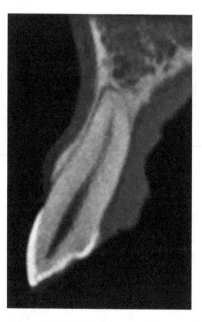

Figure 5.4 CBCT showing the difference in anatomy that occurs around anterior teeth, resulting in different injuries.

tissues, soft tissues, supporting tissues, and bone. It needs to be remembered that any tooth and its adjacent dental tissues may fit into more than one classification group, e.g. a tooth may be luxated, have a fracture extending into dentine, and be associated with a dento-alveolar fracture.

5.4 Pulp Survival/Review of Pulp Status

5.4.1 Outcomes for the Pulp

Exposure or near exposure of the pulp in the mouth and damage to the neurovascular bundle can result in one of several different outcomes for the dental pulp.

- *Pulp survival*: Minimal trauma results in the pulp surviving, relatively unchanged.
- *Localised pulp inflammation*: Exposure of the pulp in the mouth, following crown fracture, results in the surface of the exposed pulp becoming inflamed. If the site is kept clean then the inflammation

remains confined to only the superficial part of the pulp. Treatment is aimed at removing only this part of the pulp.

- *Pulp ischaemia*: This is common in luxation injuries, when the blood supply and nerve supply are affected. Teeth commonly respond negatively to pulp testing initially, but this can gradually reverse and the pulps survive by a process of revascularization and reinnervation of the pulp. This may be accompanied by transient apical breakdown, where the pulp undergoes a wound-healing response and the release of osteoclast activating factors. This causes resorption of the root-end and adjacent bone, which are seen radiographically as a widened periodontal ligament space/periapical radiolucency and apical foramen (Figure 5.5). This may persist for many months and allows the ingrowth of new blood vessels, restoring the vasculature. No intervention is required, but care needs to be taken that the radiographic findings are not mistaken for an endodontic infection.
- *Pulp obliteration*: The pulp has survived or may have undergone revascularisation

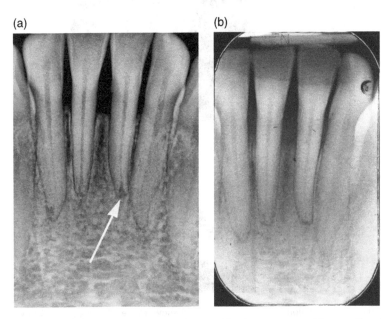

(a)　　　　　　　(b)

Figure 5.5 (a) Transient apical resorption resulting in resorption of the root tips of mandibular incisor teeth (see arrows) followed by (b) complete healing.

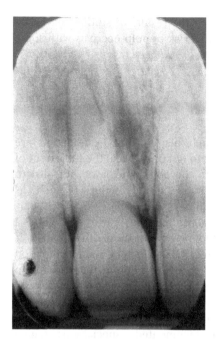

Figure 5.6 The radiographic appearance of pulp obliteration.

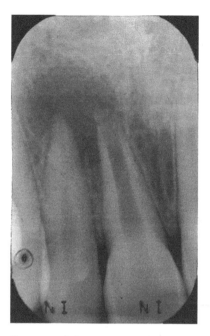

Figure 5.7 Pulp necrosis, resulting in chronic apical periodontitis, seen radiographically as a periapical radiolucency.

and has become calcified in a relatively short period of time, resulting in disappearance of the root canal, radiographically. The remaining root canal may or may not be infected (symptomatic and accompanied by radiographic signs of infection (Figure 5.6). Endodontic treatment would only be commenced if there were signs and symptoms of an endodontic infection.

- *Sterile pulp necrosis*: The blood/nerve supply to the pulp has been interrupted, but no bacteria have entered the root canal. Therefore the tooth will be asymptomatic. Root canal treatment is carried out to prevent infection and discolouration, especially if the tooth is planned to be moved orthodontically. Alternatively, a patient may choose to monitor the tooth, if the injury is classified as being at low risk of inflammatory resorption.
- *Pulp necrosis and infection*: The blood supply to the pulp has been interrupted and bacteria have infected the root canal, seen radiographically as a periapical radiolucency (Figure 5.7). Root canal treatment is indicated.

5.4.2 Different Injuries/Statistics

The more severe the injury is, the greater the risk of pulp necrosis. For minor injuries, such as enamel infraction and enamel fracture, it could be assumed that pulp necrosis would be a relatively rare event. However, rates of necrosis of 3.5% were found in one study [4] in the case of enamel infraction, which implies that other injuries, such as concussion and luxation, may also have occurred.

The rate of pulp necrosis with a number of different injuries varies with age and the stage of tooth development. In addition, pulp necrosis in cases of root fracture varies with location of the injury, mobility, and dislocation of the coronal fragment.

Figure 5.8 represents the minimum and maximum rates of pulp necrosis in hard tissue injuries.

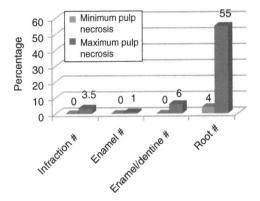

Figure 5.8 Graph showing minimum and maximum prevalence of pulp necrosis for hard tissue injuries (infraction [4,5]; enamel fracture [7,8]; enamel/dentine fracture [8,9]; root fracture [10,11]).

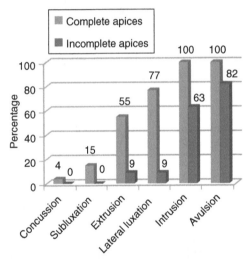

Figure 5.9 The development of pulp necrosis in luxated [12] and avulsed [13] teeth.

Figure 5.9 depicts the risk of pulp survival in fully formed teeth and for immature teeth in luxation and avulsion injuries based on clinical studies [12]. This shows the clear difference in survival when the apical foramen of the tooth is greater than 1mm wide (immature teeth).

The most severe injuries occur with avulsion and intrusion, when for teeth with complete apices the pulp necrosis rates are close to 100%.

Although the results of studies may indicate a small risk of pulp necrosis with some injuries, *teeth still need testing.*

5.5 Examination/History

A thorough history and examination are necessary to not only reveal the full extent of injuries to the teeth and jaws, but also to exclude more serious injuries, such as concussion and neck injuries, which may need urgent medical care. Although a detailed knowledge of these other injuries is not needed, a basic history and examination to exclude them are required. Questioning an accompanying person may also be necessary if recollection of events is not clear. The history and examination must be thorough and well documented, especially as trauma is a common cause for medico-legal action.

5.5.1 History

Important questions to ask when a patient presents after dental trauma include:

- Apart from the damage to teeth and jaws, did you experience a loss of consciousness, nausea, vomiting, amnesia, or headache? If the answer is yes, have you sought medical assistance?
- Did you sustain any other injuries or do you have any symptoms from other parts of your body?
- When did the injury occur? Important with respect to treatment planning, e.g. the time an avulsed tooth has been out of its socket/kept dry and subsequently prognosis of injuries. A delay in seeking treatment may indicate a non-accidental injury.
- Where did it happen? Important with regards to tetanus prophylaxis.
- How did it happen? This may give an indication of what injuries to expect in the oral region as well as elsewhere in the body.
- Do you have or have you had any pain? If the answer is yes, then a pain history is required, which can be remembered by

the acronym SOCRATES (**S**ite, **O**nset, **C**haracter, **R**adiation, **A**ssociations, **T**ime course, **E**xacerbating/Relieving factors, **S**everity).

- Any history of previous injuries or recent dental treatment? Certain athletes may be prone to repeated injuries, and a history and examination may reveal these findings to be historic and not needing treatment.
- Have you had any treatment already? This also includes first aid given at a sporting event, e.g. timing of reimplantation of a tooth and storage medium.
- Have all avulsed teeth or teeth fragments been accounted for? If not and if there is a possibility that they have been swallowed or inhaled, then a chest/abdominal radio-graph needs to be taken to exclude this.
- If a tooth was avulsed, how long was it out of the socket and how was it stored?
- Did any teeth move and can you bite together as you did previously? As well as identifying luxated teeth interfering with the occlusion, this may help identify minor or major fracture of the jaws.

When questioning a patient, problems of memory and the manner in which answers are given may indicate a head injury.

5.5.2   Medical History

A standard medical history is required to identify any medical conditions that may modify the approach to treatment, e.g. allergy to latex. In addition, tetanus status should be determined as additional prophylaxis may be required. An immunisation programme has been in place in the UK since 1961 and in other parts of the world for a similar period of time. However, some athletes may not have received some or the entire vaccination schedule. Also, the vaccines available in some countries may not offer the same degree of protection against all the antigens used in the vaccines of other countries. Therefore this must be checked, as a booster injection of tetanus immunoglobulin is easy to arrange, whereas the consequences of not protecting against this disease can include death.

5.5.3   Full Examination

A thorough, systematic examination is required, starting extra-orally, moving intra-orally, and then focusing on the teeth and adjacent soft tissues. Athletes with injuries often attend hospital prior to any dental assessment. However, it is still necessary to not just focus on teeth, as injuries can be missed and damage distant from the teeth may still need treatment and give clues to dental injuries.

Extra-oral examination should start with soft tissue examination, looking for cuts and bruising, which may be superficial or indicate deeper injuries. The jaws should be palpated, feeling for irregularities and painful areas, which may indicate bony fractures. Lips are commonly damaged and may contain tooth fragments if lacerations are present.

Intra-oral examination is started in a similar way. Any blood clots should be removed using saline prior to examination, then soft tissues should be investigated for lacerations, abrasions, and bruising, and the jaws thoroughly palpated, looking for irregularities and painful areas.

The patient's occlusion should be checked to make sure that opposing teeth contact in a similar way to that prior to the injury taking place. This should be confirmed by the patient. A malocclusion or interfering tooth may indicate a jaw fracture, or fractured/lux-ated teeth.

5.5.4   Tooth-specific Examination

It is rare for only a single tooth to be trauma-tised, due to the size of most striking objects being relatively large. Therefore the site of the traumatic impact should be located and then adjacent teeth and opposing teeth should be examined. The following tests should be performed:

- Teeth should be percussed lightly with a dental mirror, their crowns pressed and their adjacent soft tissues palpated to test for inflammation (pain), which indicates damage to the periodontal tissues.

(a)

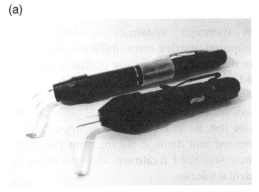

(b)

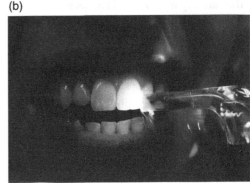

Figure 5.10 A bore light (a) can be used to transilluminate teeth, when looking for infraction lines, and is covered with a clear plastic shield (b) for cross-infection purposes.

- While percussing teeth, a high-pitched ringing sound produced as the tooth is struck may indicate ankylosis. Although this doesn't normally occur until roughly a month after a severe injury, it may be present from a *previous* injury. It is important medico-legally to record that this has occurred due to a previous injury rather than the most recent one.
- Teeth should be inspected for:
  - Infraction lines (incomplete fractures confined to enamel). These are best viewed using a fibre optic light directed as close to 90° to the fracture line as possible. A relatively cheap option is to use a bore light (Figure 5.10a), covered in a protective plastic shield for cross-infection purposes (Figure 5.10b), which is normally used to inspect gun barrels.
  - Fractures and whether these are confined to enamel, dentine, the crown and root, or just the root of a tooth (Figure 5.11).
  - Pulp exposure, in the case of complicated crown and crown–root fractures (Figure 5.12).
  - Displacement, indicating a luxation or fracture injury (Figure 5.13).
  - Colour changes. These may indicate bleeding into the pulp in luxation injuries (pink), and then the breakdown of blood products in the pulp (blue/purple), both of which may be reversible changes. Pulp necrosis (grey/black) or

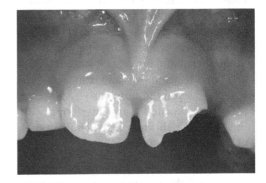

Figure 5.11 A fractured crown of a permanent central incisor.

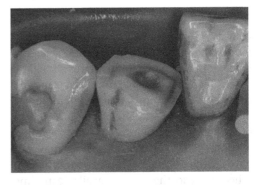

Figure 5.12 Pulp exposure, following a crown fracture.

pulp obliteration occurring sometime after an injury (yellow) can also be seen (Figure 5.14a–c). No colour changes are seen when teeth are uninjured or in severe injuries initially, when blood vessels are completely severed.

- Mobility of teeth should be assessed. The commonest classification is as follows [14]:
  - Class I is tooth movement in a bucco-lingual or mesio-distal direction < 1 mm

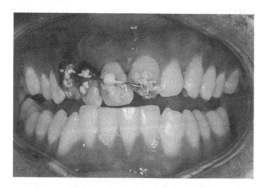

Figure 5.13 Luxated right maxillary incisors which have been poorly splinted. Note their lower position when compared to the contra-lateral teeth.

- Class II > 1 mm, but no vertical movement
- Class III > 1 mm and mobility of the tooth vertically.

Loose teeth may be due to a luxation injury or fracture of teeth/bone.

- Pain from the patient's gingivae with a non-painful stimulus (allodynia) should be assessed by lightly touching the gingivae with a cotton bud. This may indicate neuropathic pain if it remains following the healing of tissues and endodontic infections.

5.5.5 Radiographs

The types of radiographs required will be determined following the history and clinical examination. More extensive injuries may need extra-oral views, such as a panoramic view, to detect fractures of the jaws.

(a)

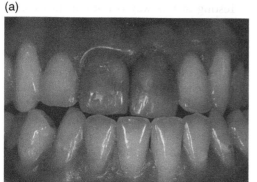

(b)

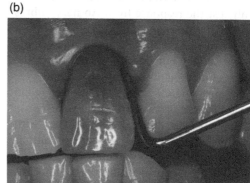

(c)

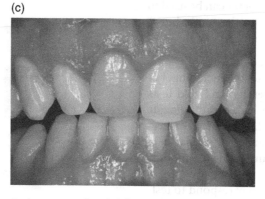

Figure 5.14 Colour changes in the crowns of teeth following luxation (a), after pulp necrosis (b) and root canal obliteration (c).

For intra-oral injuries, current guidelines recommend the following:

- A periapical radiograph, taken with the film parallel to the teeth and the central x-ray beam aimed at 90° to both
- An occlusal view
- A periapical radiograph directed from the mesial or distal aspect of the tooth in question.

The purpose of exposing radiographs at different angles to the central x-ray beam is to identify injuries such as root fractures, which may only be visible when the beam passes within 15–20° of the fracture line, which may be at an oblique angle rather than horizontally directed.

5.5.6 Pulp Testing

Testing the dental pulp, to assess that it is healthy, is normally performed using thermal testing or electrical testing. However, these only test the response from Aδ nerve fibres within the pulp and not the blood supply. A positive response indicates a functioning nerve supply, but doesn't indicate that the pulp is inflammation-free.

Because reinnervation is slower than revascularization, an initial negative response to pulp testing should be interpreted with caution, unless there are clear indications that the pulp has died, e.g. following avulsion of a completely formed tooth or when signs and symptoms indicate the presence of infection. Laser Doppler flowmetry can be used to assess the blood supply to the tooth, but is rarely used in clinical practice.

- *Thermal tests*: A variety of ways of testing have been used on teeth, including hot tests (heated gutta percha) and cold tests (ethyl chloride, Endo-Ice®, carbon dioxide snow). Due to its availability and temperature (−27 °C), Endo-Ice® or a similar cold refrigerant spray (Figure 5.15) is commonly used in dental surgeries, as even teeth restored with crowns may respond to testing. A cotton bud or cotton pellet is soaked in the liquid, which is then applied to the

tooth. One slight drawback that has been recognised is that both this and carbon dioxide snow may be associated with the development of infraction lines on teeth.

- *Electric pulp tester*: There are a number of these on the market, but they all work on the same principle, that of a gradually increasing voltage at its tip. Teeth are dried and isolated (using acetate strips between teeth), then the tip is applied to the tooth near to its incisal edge, using a small amount of toothpaste to aid conduction of the electrical current (Figure 5.16a). The lip hook attached to the pulp tester is held in the patient's hand to complete the circuit (Figure 5.16b). The patient is told to let go of the hook when they feel a similar sensation to that of a non-traumatised tooth, used as a reference. Exposed enamel must be present to test teeth, avoiding testing of crowned teeth at their gingival margins.

Testing in this way is not conclusive and needs to be used in combination with other signs and symptoms. When teeth are sore, it is common for patients to respond positively to a test due to pressure from either the cotton pellet or pulp tester probe. It should be made clear to the patient what they are meant to feel by performing on an injured tooth first. If still in doubt, then the cotton bud can be used without Endo-Ice and the pulp tester disconnected to test the reliability of the patient's response.

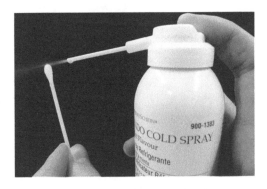

Figure 5.15 A cold refrigerant spray, used to thermally test the pulps of teeth.

(a)   (b)

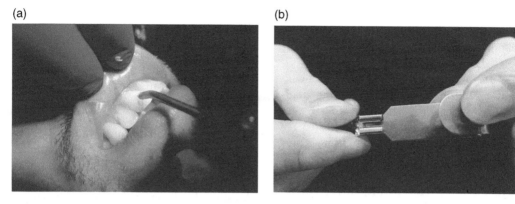

Figure 5.16 An electric pulp tester used on an isolated tooth (a) and the patient holding the lip hook to complete the electrical circuit (b).

5.6   Treatment

5.6.1   Preventive Measures to Maintain Pulp Health

Mouth guards/face masks/helmets: Prevention is always better than cure and wearing protective equipment can reduce the number of injuries sustained to teeth and therefore the risk of pulp damage. At a tooth level, fractures and displacement are reduced. Please see Chapter 7.

5.6.2   Emergency Treatment: Protection of Dentine

At an emergency appointment, which can often be stressful, it is easy to forget to protect exposed dentine following crown fractures when teeth have to be reimplanted or repositioned. The exposed dentine is different to that exposed during tooth surface loss, as even minor trauma may impair the blood supply to the pulp. Following this the outward flow of dentinal fluid though the exposed tubules may reduce or even stop completely. This can allow bacteria to invade the exposed tubules on the fractured dentine surface, which eventually causes pulp necrosis. An attempt should be made to protect all exposed dentine with either dentine-bonded composite or glass ionomer.

In younger patients, crown fractures often extend sub-gingivally due to teeth not being

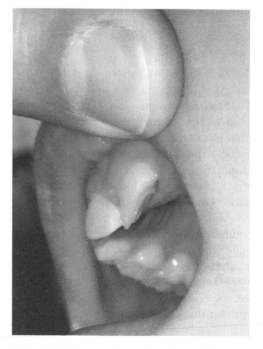

Figure 5.17 A crown fracture in a 9-year-old, showing its sub-gingival nature due to the crown not being fully erupted.

fully erupted (Figures 5.11 and 5.17). Attempts at dentine bonding may be unsuccessful due to problems with moisture control at the sub-gingival margin. Following the control of any bleeding, glass ionomer can be used as a temporary material on the palatal aspect of teeth, as bonding is easier to achieve using this material. The labial aspect and incisal edge can be restored with composite. When the tooth is fully erupted, the glass ionomer can be replaced with dentine-bonded composite.

Sealing of enamel and dentine cracks with light-cured unfilled resin, following acid-etching of enamel, appeared to prevent bacterial invasion of teeth in an in-vitro model [15], but failed to prevent it in a simulated animal model [16], which more closely represented what happens in humans. There are a number of reasons why this treatment may not have worked, but exposed dentine at the cervical margin of teeth is an alternative pathway of infection that would not be blocked by coating only the enamel of teeth.

5.6.3 Periodontal Disease

The periodontal health of dental trauma patients is often overlooked. It becomes more of an issue in adults who may have more advanced periodontal disease, where root surfaces of teeth have become coated with plaque. If the pulps in these teeth are compromised, then the bacteria coating the roots have a better chance of infecting the pulp space. Therefore, oral hygiene instruction and even basic periodontal treatment may be required at the patient's emergency visit to reduce the chance of infection. Using a 0.2% chlorhexidine mouthwash for the first week after trauma helps to prevent plaque formation, especially when the mouth is sore and tooth brushing is difficult.

5.6.4 Wet Storage > 5 Minutes/Dry Storage

Current guidelines urge the reimplantation of avulsed teeth as soon as possible. It has been shown that pulp survival decreases when the time of wet storage of avulsed teeth exceeds 5 minutes [17]. Dry storage of teeth is a disaster in relation to pulp survival. Therefore, prompt reimplantation continues to be one of the most important factors in pulps surviving in immature teeth that have been avulsed.

5.6.5 Treatment of Avulsed Teeth with Tetracyclines

In addition to reimplanting teeth quickly, it has been shown that a doxycycline solution applied to teeth can double the rate of pulp survival [18]. The solution is made from 1 mg of doxycycline in 20 ml of saline and the tooth is soaked in it for 5 minutes. This improvement only occurred with the local application of the drug and not when given systemically [19]. Alternatively, minocycline (Arestin™) has been used. This has been used on teeth for the same time period, to further increase the chance of revascularization [20]. A more recent, retrospective human study showed no benefit when using topical doxycycline [21], which may relate to the differences between experimental animal studies and human studies.

5.6.6 Root Fractures: Optimal Repositioning and Splinting Type

When looking at pulp survival in root fractured teeth, research has shown that the optimal positioning of the fractured portion and use of a flexible splint improve pulp survival when compared to poor repositioning and rigid (cap) splints [22].

5.6.7 Vital Pulp Treatment

When pulps become exposed or nearly exposed following crown fracture, the pulp needs to be preserved or removed, depending on its status and the importance of preserving it to allow the completion of tooth formation. All attempts should be made to preserve the pulp, especially when its removal and replacement with a root filling leaves a thin-walled tooth, prone to fracture.

The approach to management depends on the time elapsed after the crown facture and the depth of the fracture (whether the pulp is exposed), as the aim of treatment is to prevent necrosis of the pulp. Younger patients with dentine containing wide dentinal tubules and concomitant luxation injuries affecting the blood supply to the pulp, may pose further risks to the pulp's health.

If the pulp is unexposed then the tooth should be isolated under local anaesthetic, cleaned and disinfected with 2.5% sodium hypochlorite and then rinsed with saline, to remove any bacteria. The pulp should be capped with calcium hydroxide and the tooth restored with glass ionomer and dentine-bonded composite. Calcium hydroxide causes the release of growth factors within the dentine matrix which stimulate the formation of reparative dentine around the nearly exposed pulp.

If the pulp is exposed, then a decision needs to be made about what treatment to perform:

1) Based on one of a number of animal studies [23], direct pulp capping is generally indicated in teeth with small exposures, treated shortly after injury (within 24 hours). The surrounding dentine needs to be disinfected with 2.5% sodium hypochlorite and then rinsed with saline. Hard-setting or non-setting calcium hydroxide can then be placed over the pulp and the tooth restored with a covering of glass ionomer and dentine-bonded composite.

2) Partial pulpotomy is indicated when only the superficial part of the exposed pulp is inflamed and the underlying pulp is healthy. In anterior teeth with pulps exposed by dental trauma, the cleansing effect of saliva and oral hygiene measures limit plaque build-up near the pulp. In an animal study [24], it was found that the extent of the inflammation was limited to the most superficial part of the pulp, extending 2 mm deep, when the exposure was present for seven days or less. A clinical study by the same author [25] showed that partial pulpotomies had a success rate of 96% and this appeared to be unaffected by the time or the size of pulp exposure, if this was less than 4 mm^2. However, although the time from exposure of the pulp to treatment was as long as 90 days, the vast majority of teeth were treated within five days. A recent review [26] looking at the success rate of partial pulpotomies showed that a delay of treatment of less than nine days had a minimal effect on the outcome.

The fracture site needs to be cleaned with 2.5% sodium hypochlorite or a chlorhexidine solution to ensure it is bacteria-free. To perform a partial pulpotomy, the most suitable instrument is a diamond bur in a turbine handpiece, cooled with saline. The diamond bur should be a similar size to the pulp exposure. Ideally, a turbine handpiece such as the Impact Air 45° handpiece (Figure 5.18) should be used, as this vents its air away from the pulpotomy site, preventing contamination with oil lubricant. The bur should extend up to 2 mm below the site of exposure, severing the most coronal part of the pulp.

The pulp is rinsed with saline and then observed to see that the bleeding stops (Figure 5.19a), which indicates the pulp has been amputated to a level where inflammation is not present. If bleeding continues then the pulp needs amputating at a lower level. The wound site is dried, and then calcium hydroxide powder mixed with sterile water is applied as a thick paste into the cavity (Figure 5.19b). Excess moisture can be removed using cotton pellets, gently packing the calcium hydroxide into the cavity. Any excess should be removed, the walls of the cavity cleaned, and the rest of the cavity filled with zinc oxide/eugenol (Figure 5.19c) such as intermediate restorative material (IRM°).

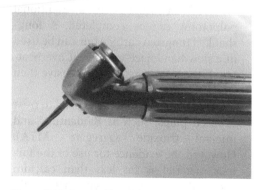

Figure 5.18 Impact Air 45° handpiece.

(a) (b)

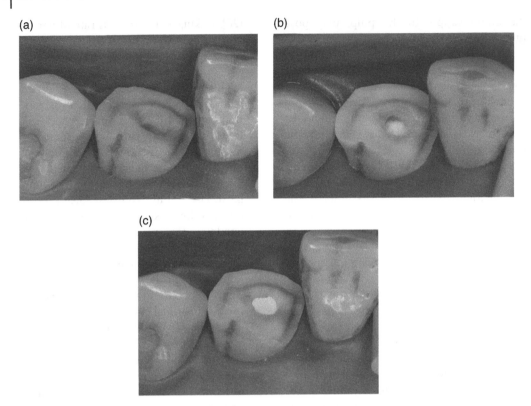

(c)

Figure 5.19 A partial pulpotomy, following pulp amputation and haemostasis (a), application of calcium hydroxide (b) and sealing with IRM® (c).

This can be covered with glass ionomer and then the remaining tooth built up with dentine-bonded composite. Creating a 2-mm deep cavity makes sealing the pulp a lot easier.

If bleeding continues following amputation of the pulp, then further pulp tissue needs removing until bleeding stops. This may result in all of the coronal pulp being removed, in which case a traditional pulpotomy can be completed. A long-shanked tungsten carbide bur can be used in a slow handpiece to prevent overheating. If the inflammation is extensive then a pulpectomy may be indicated.

Other materials have been used to treat exposed pulps, such as Biodentine® and mineral trioxide aggregate (MTA). However, the evidence for use of the former material is far less than calcium hydroxide, while conventional MTA stains dentine.

5.6.8 Endodontic Treatment

The pulp may be damaged following trauma due to direct physical damage to its nerve/ blood supply, exposure to the oral cavity following the fracture or cracking of dentine and enamel, and then contamination with bacteria from the mouth. Physical damage may only be prevented by minimising the chance/extent of damage, e.g. using a mouth guard, while bacterial contamination is prevented by prompt coverage of exposed dentine with a suitable restoration and vital pulp therapy if indicated. Failure to prevent either of these may lead to root canal treatment being required.

5.6.8.1 Role of Bacteria

The role of bacteria in the development of apical periodontitis was demonstrated in 1965 [27]. Other causes/associations have also been identified, including bacterial products, viruses, fungi, and archaea, but the role of some of these may be limited. It is the interaction of bacteria and their products, and the host that is responsible for the disease process. The host's inflammatory and immune responses act together to try and defend the body from the bacteria, and the resulting accumulation of defence cells and inflammatory mediators start the process of bone resorption at the tooth's apex. This is seen radiographically as a periapical radiolucency. Due to the isolation and hence survival of the bacteria in the root canal from the host's defences, the inflammation becomes chronic. This is characterised by the presence of inflammation and attempts at healing at the same time.

From this point the initial lesion may remain in this chronic state or become acute (including suppuration in both cases), progressing to an abscess or cyst formation. The aim of endodontic treatment is to prevent or treat these conditions.

5.6.8.2 Success

The success of root canal treatment varies [28], depending on whether a tooth is vital (90.7%), a periapical radiolucency is absent (92.5%), present (75.6%), if it is primary treatment (83%), or if root canal retreatment (80%) is required. Even the success of surgery can vary, depending on whether traditional techniques (59%) or micro-surgery (94%) are employed [29]. This doesn't mean that all teeth are best treated immediately following trauma to obtain the highest success rates, as the pulps in many of the teeth will survive.

Luxated teeth that have received mild and moderate injuries provide diagnostic challenges, as many teeth initially respond negatively to pulp testing. However, they are at a low risk of inflammatory root resorption compared to injuries such as avulsion and intrusion. Therefore a 'wait and see' approach can be taken.

Those that eventually develop root canal obliteration present technical challenges when locating their root canals and then ensuring that the whole root canal is disinfected without the original canal being transported or blocked at any point. They should not be prospectively root treated to make treatment more straightforward without clear signs and symptoms of endodontic infection being present. Only a proportion of the pulps become necrotic: 27.2% [30] or less. A skilled operator should be able to locate and negotiate an obliterated root canal, and anterior teeth are relatively easy to disinfect (as opposed to the more complex anatomy found in posterior teeth). Anterior teeth are also more amenable to surgical treatment, if required.

Prospectively root-treating teeth will lead to many unnecessary treatments being completed, often on teeth that are thin-walled (incompletely developed teeth that have been traumatised are much more prone to root canal obliteration).

However, initial treatment should be performed to as high a standard as possible to ensure the best chance of it producing a successful outcome.

5.6.8.3 Rubber Dam

Rubber dam, despite being used in dentistry for over 150 years, is rarely used in general practice. It has obvious benefits, such as improving access to the tooth, moisture control and preventing contamination of the root canal and the dentist. Even though there is limited evidence to show that root canal treatment under rubber dam isolation is more successful, preventing the swallowing or inhalation of instruments and irrigants is justification for its use, alone.

There are a number of different materials and techniques to isolate teeth, but the following way is suggested as an easy method:

- Prior to its application, floss the teeth to check inter-proximal contacts are clear and also to remove plaque that may be pushed sub-gingivally into healing wounds. Teeth should also be cleaned labially and palatally/lingually if plaque is present.

(a)

(b)

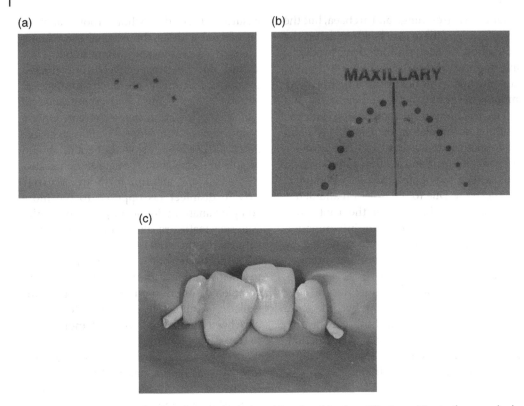

(c)

Figure 5.20 The position of teeth, when marked on a rubber dam (a), often differ in position to those marked with a stamp (b). Marking the true positions on the dam make placement straightforward (c).

- Use 150 mm × 150 mm heavy gauge (0.3 mm thick) latex, or a non-latex variety.
- When punching holes, mark the location of each tooth on the dam rather than estimating teeth location or using a standard ink stamp (Figure 5.20a–c).
- The largest punched holes on the rubber dam punch are suitable for most teeth.
- Rubber Wedjets can be placed between teeth to retain the dam. If the teeth are spaced, the dam can be retained with a clamp (IVORY #00, IVORY #6, IVORY #9, IVORY #9S, IVORY #212 or IVORY #212SA).
- When using a clamp, one hole for each tooth requiring treatment is sufficient. When using Wedjets, a single hole per tooth is sufficient, but an adjacent tooth either side gives better access.
- If a splint is still present and needs to remain in place, then the tooth can be

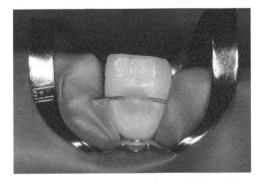

Figure 5.21 Placement of rubber dam when a splint is still attached to teeth, using an IVORY #9 clamp.

clamped with an IVORY #9, as shown in Figure 5.21, though there will be gaps between the rubber dam and the tooth between the splint and the clamp. These must be filled (see below) to prevent the ingress of saliva. A lubricant, such as shaving cream or Vaseline, may be applied to the teeth to allow the dam to pass the contacts points more easily.

- If a clamp is used, always attach a length of floss to prevent it being swallowed or inhaled.
- Ensure the rubber dam has been everted (tucked into the gingival crevice). If a tooth has been avulsed and root canal treatment is starting 7–10 days later, then avoid pushing the dam sub-gingivally to prevent damage to the healing periodontal tissues.
- Any deficiencies around the dam should be filled with Oraseal®.
- Disinfect the tooth and adjacent dam with 2.5% sodium hypochlorite prior to accessing the tooth, to reduce the chance of contamination of the root canal.

5.6.8.4 Instrumentation

Traumatised teeth requiring root canal treatment can present a number of problems to the clinician, e.g. locating the root canal in teeth with obliterated pulps and knowing how far to instrument in root-fractured teeth. However, the principles behind treatment are similar to teeth that haven't been traumatised.

Treatment is based on the prevention of formation, or the elimination of the existing bacteria biofilm and bacterial products in a root canal. A combination of mechanical preparation and chemical disinfection aims to clean the root canal. However, in practice, sterilisation of the root canal is not possible due to the complexity of the root canal and the difficulty in instrumenting and delivering a suitable irrigant to all parts of it. This is a similar situation to the treatment of periodontal disease, where a bacterial biofilm on the outside of the tooth is removed to the best of a clinician's ability, but where again sterilisation isn't possible. In both cases, the combination of mechanical instrumentation and disinfection reduces the contamination to a level compatible with healing.

Mechanical preparation improves access to the root canal system for the chemical disinfection as well as creating a shape that is easy to eventually fill. It also removes some of

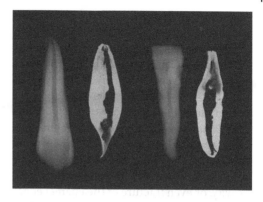

Figure 5.22 Radiographic images compared to actual anatomy, seen when root canals are stained and then cleared in a maxillary lateral incisor (left) and mandibular lateral incisor (right).

the biofilm and infected dentine. Even relatively straight-looking root canals can be more complex than they first seem (Figure 5.22). The debris produced, along with the remains of the pulp, can then be flushed away with a suitable irrigant, whose disinfectant properties help to remove the majority of the remaining infection. The greater the mechanical preparation, the more effective the chemical disinfection is, due to greater penetration of irrigant. However, there is a balance between dentine removal and weakening of the remaining tooth structure; therefore the minimum amount of dentine should be removed from the tooth to facilitate the disinfection process.

- *Access*: Penetration into the tooth through enamel or porcelain (if an indirect restoration in the form of a crown is present), is performed using a diamond burr, followed by a tungsten carbide burr to penetrate the dentine and then into the pulp chamber. The roof of the pulp chamber can then be removed. The final shape of the access cavity will be determined by the shape of the pulp chamber. Therefore, although every access cavity may have a similar shape for each tooth type, their size and location will vary. Straight-line access has been suggested to allow better mechanical instrumentation of the canal walls, to allow deeper penetration of irrigant and to reduce the stress on instruments. However, in anterior teeth, the need for this is not as great as the canals are often fairly wide and straight anyway, especially in the young. Straight-line access in this situation will often mean the access cavity extends onto the labial surface of the tooth or through the incisal edge. This can result in poor aesthetics long-term due to staining of the composite resin used to restore the access cavity, or even fracture of the enamel edge. Even straight-line access does not allow instrumentation of all parts of the canal wall [31], which is compounded by complex anatomy that is sometimes present. A better option is to locate the access cavity slightly palatal to the incisal edge, which preserves aesthetics but allows almost straight-line access to the root canal (Figure 5.23).

- *Types of instrumentation for anterior teeth*: There are a variety of instruments for preparing root canals. Despite advances in instrument technology, there have been no improvements in the success rates of endodontic treatment over the past 40–50 years. It is beyond the scope of this chapter to review all of them; clinicians should use whatever technique they are comfortable with. However, due to preparation of the root canals in anterior teeth being relatively easy to perform, the vast

majority can be completed using hand instruments such as Hedstrom files, Flex-o-Files, and Gates Glidden burs (Figure 5.24).

- *Instrumentation technique*: The aims when preparing a root canal are to produce a shape that is large enough to allow disinfection and allows the easy placement of the final root filling, providing some resistance to pushing it through the apical foramen. The only way to achieve this with conventional instruments is to produce a tapered preparation, from the widest point (access cavity) to the narrowest point (root end). The extent to which this is needed depends on the initial size of the root canal. Fine root canals need greater preparation to achieve these aims, and the final shape will be largely determined by the operator. Wide canals may need little or no preparation, as their shapes may already be sufficiently wide to disinfect and fill, and further preparation will serve little purpose and may even weaken the teeth. The exact preparation can be determined by the initial canal shape/size.

For a relatively straight root canal in an anterior tooth, the preparation at the apical foramen should be a minimum of size 30 (0.3 mm diameter). The rationale for this is that a 27 gauge endodontic syringe needle, which has a diameter of 0.41 mm, will fit within 2 mm of the end of the root

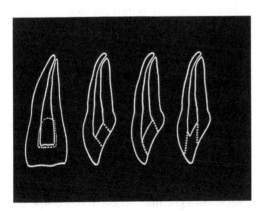

Figure 5.23 From the left, an access cavity when seen palatally, prepared through the cingulum, with a balanced preparation, and straight-line access.

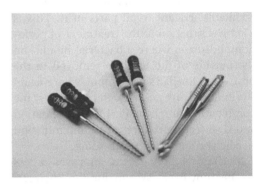

Figure 5.24 Hedstrom files, Flex-o-Files, and Gates Glidden burrs are often the only instruments required for root canal preparation.

(a)

(b)

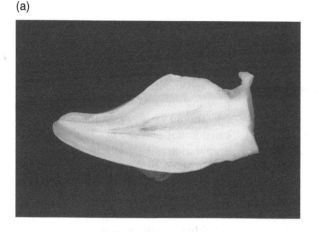
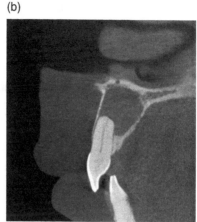

Figure 5.25 An obliterated root canal can sometimes extend a good distance coronally (a) as well as being patent throughout its whole length and curved apically (b).

canal and allow sufficient exchange of irrigant when combined with patency filing, recapitulation of instruments, and some form of active irrigation, if possible. Based on this, there are several ways to prepare the tooth:

- *Narrow root canal*: it will be difficult to negotiate initially and the vast majority of the canal will need preparing. In single-rooted maxillary incisors, the root canals are always located in the centre of the tooth. Experience and a good sense of spatial awareness are required to locate the canal, which may extend some distance coronally (Figure 5.25a). CBCT scans help in their localization and also reveal that root canals are often patent throughout their length and wider (in their labio-palatal dimension) than the root canal seen on a conventional radiograph (Figure 5.25b). Curvatures in the root canal often occur apically and are also seen (Figure 5.25b). This insight may prevent ledging of the outer aspect of the root canal wall, which is very easy to do with an instrument that is not pre-curved, due to the relatively soft nature of the tertiary dentine.

- *Moderate-sized root canal*: narrower parts of the canal (apically) will need preparation, but the more coronal

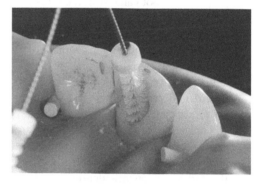

Figure 5.26 Sterile interdental brushes, used to clean wide root canals.

portion may be so wide in diameter that even the largest instruments are loose when preparing the canal at that length. In this case, these portions of the canal walls should be brushed to remove any biofilm present, preserving as much dentine as possible.

- *Large root canal*: little if any preparation is required, as the walls of the tooth are thin and prone to fracture long term. It is also necessary to leave a portion of the pulp chamber roof intact, as extending this to eliminate the roof will remove a significant amount of dentine and weaken the tooth. The root canal can be cleaned with sterile, interdental brushes (Figure 5.26) and any remaining pulp chamber roof or pulp horns cleaned with a curved ultrasonic tip. When using the brushes, it is advisable to use these initially then rely on the irrigant alone to disinfect the canal. Extrusion of sodium hypochlorite is a possibility if the root canal is filled with irrigant then the brush rapidly pushed down. To minimise this, after irrigation, the sodium hypochlorite can be removed using a second syringe before inserting the brush slowly to brush the walls. This sequence can then be repeated. This technique is often used in root fractured teeth and teeth with incompletely formed apices, which have wide root canals and large apical foramina.

There are a variety of techniques to prepare the root canal with hand instruments, including: step back, step down, crown down, etc. As well as this, the method of manipulating instruments can involve filing, watch-winding, or a balanced force technique. One way (step down) is detailed below. The sequence for rotary instruments is similar, but they will only prepare the canals when they are relatively narrow, which is less frequent in anterior teeth than posterior teeth. In fact they may not engage dentine at all in anterior teeth in the young. Readers are advised to read manufacturers' instructions regarding their exact sequence as a number of systems now exist.

Suggested technique:

- Use a pre-operative radiograph to assess root canal anatomy.
- Prepare the access cavity as suggested previously, using tungsten carbide #256 and Endo-Z burs.
- Ensure irrigant is introduced into the root canal.
- Explore the root canal shape with a 08 Flex-O-File.
- Prepare the coronal portion of the canal using Hedstrom files (15–40), filing circumferentially.

If resistance is met, then it may imply there is a curve in the sagittal plane which is not apparent from the pre-operative radiograph. Do not file beyond this curve, if present.

- Irrigant should be used between each new instrument. An 08 or 10 Flex-O-File should be used to make sure the canal is not blocked below the coronal preparation. Gentle insertion will loosen any debris.
- Use an 08 or 10 Flex-O-File to establish patency.
- Determine the working length using a suitably sized file and apex locator, and take a radiograph to confirm this.
- Reduce the working length from 0.5 mm to 1.0 mm short of the '0' value and use this length as the final working length.
- Insert the largest file that first binds at full working length and use a filing, stem-winding or balanced force technique, preparing the tooth till the next largest instrument reaches the working length. If there is difficulty in manipulating the instrument, then continue preparation with a smaller one.
- Use an 08 or 10 file to check patency.
- Repeat with the next largest file and so on till a minimum size of 30 is reached. Most anterior root canals will be larger than this size at their apices. In this case, prepare the root canal to a file size that just starts to cut dentine at its tip (seen by dentine shavings collecting on the file).
- A step-back technique can then be used. The next largest file is used to prepare the root canal, 1 mm shorter than the last file. Following irrigation and patency filing, this is then repeated a further 1 mm shorter and so on, till the root canal has a uniform taper. The exact taper will depend on the original size of the root canal. If the root canal is wide, a 010 taper may be necessary. If greater still, then the canal should not be enlarged any further, as irrigation

and obturation should be easy to accomplish. Once the canal reaches a size much greater than the largest endodontic instruments available, then brushes should be used to clean the canal walls in combination with sodium hypochlorite.

- *Root-fractured teeth*: Pulps in teeth with root fractures often survive. If emergency treatment is successful then hard tissue healing can occur, where the two portions of teeth join together via a hard callus of cementum and dentine, which unites the two separate pieces. If the pulp remains healthy then no further treatment is required.

If the pulp becomes necrotic, then root canal treatment is indicated. The tooth is instrumented, irrigated, and filled up to the fracture line (Figure 5.27). The pulp in the apical portion often survives and can be left.

If the pulp survives, but hard tissue repair doesn't occur, then the tooth can often be left as long as there is no

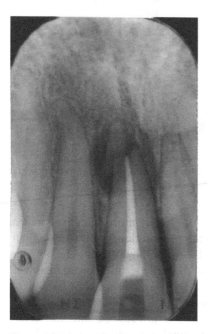

Figure 5.27 In root-fractured teeth, instrumentation and obturation are completed up to the fracture line.

discomfort on eating. If the fracture line is located coronally then pressure on the crown will often produce pain due to pulp stimulation when the crown moves. In this case one of the following options can be chosen to reduce or eliminate the pain:

- Monitor the tooth as the root canal in the coronal portion will gradually obliterate, reducing the discomfort felt.
- Splint the coronal portion to the adjacent teeth with a lingual or palatal retainer wire, providing there is space to fit the wire (Figure 5.28).
- Root fill the coronal portion. This rarely needs to be done.

5.6.8.5 Choice of Irrigant

The gold standard for irrigation is sodium hypochlorite. The exact strength used in most studies has ranged between 0.5 and 5%, obtaining high success rates, but a 2.5% solution is perfectly adequate to dissolve organic tissue, kill bacteria, and lubricate instruments used. What is important is to frequently replenish it within the root canal, using a side-vented needle and syringe to deliver it, reducing the risk of a hypochlorite accident. A penultimate rinse of 17% EDTA can be used to remove the smear layer generated during mechanical preparation and helps to degrade any remaining biofilm.

There are a variety of ways of improving the effect of irrigation. Irrigant will only be effective if it is completely replenished by introducing fresh solution. It is only replenished close to the tip of the syringe needle, depending on its exact design. Therefore a thinner needle tip (30 gauge) should be used to increase the depth of irrigant delivery. It should be remembered that root canals in anterior teeth are often slightly curved in a labio-palatal direction, therefore the irrigation needle should also be curved to negotiate the full length of the root canal.

The irrigant beyond the needle that stays stagnant can be replenished by recapitulation, which involves inserting a small file to length

(a)

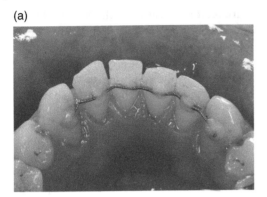

(b)

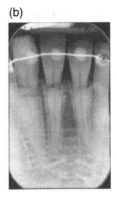

Figure 5.28 Several root-fractured teeth reviewed five years after trauma, immobilised with a wire splint (a) and with healthy pulps (b), despite the accumulation of calculus.

and moving it up and down. This disperses the suspension of dentine in the apical portion into the more coronal part of the root canal, allowing its removal. Patency filing, which involves passing a small file (size 08 or 10) 0.5–1 mm beyond the apical foramen, prevents debris from getting compacted apically.

A simple way to improve irrigation of the apical portion of the root canal following mechanical preparation is by using a customised gutta percha point in a pumping action, which results in active irrigation, as opposed to passive irrigation when just using an endodontic syringe alone. A 04 taper cone that is slightly larger than the apical preparation is customised by dipping its tip in chloroform for a second, then inserting it to length into the root canal. It is then used in a pumping action, with a vertical movement of 5 mm, inserting then removing the cone twice every second.

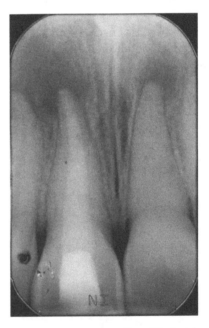

Figure 5.29 A dense, uniform fill of calcium hydroxide, introduced with an amalgam carrier and packed with pluggers.

5.6.8.6 Inter-appointment Dressings

If treatment is completed over several visits then a dressing of calcium hydroxide should be used as in inter-appointment dressing. It is effective at preventing or treating external inflammatory resorption, as well as helping to control existing infection. It comes in various preparations, but is most effective when the proportion of calcium hydroxide is highest. Therefore calcium hydroxide powder, made radiopaque by the addition of barium

sulfate (ratio 7:1) is more effective than a commercial preparation, where less than 50% may be calcium hydroxide. The powder is mixed with sterile water and can be introduced into the root canal using files, or a spiral filler. In wide canals, a thicker mix is prepared and is introduced into the canal using an amalgam carrier followed by packing of the material, using a plugger (Figure 5.29).

5.6.8.7 Obturation

Obturation of the root canals in anterior teeth is normally straightforward. The aim is to fill the root canals three-dimensionally using a filling material and sealer, to prevent (re)contamination after they have been cleaned, shaped, and disinfected. There are a variety of techniques to fill the root canal, the details of which are beyond the scope of this chapter. However, they all have to fulfil certain requirements, which will be described in relation to the lateral compaction technique:

- The root filling should reach to the end of the prepared root canal. This is easy to achieve in anterior teeth by measuring the length of gutta percha points and ensuring they reach to the full length of the canal or to where the finger spreader last reached.
- Gutta percha points should be disinfected in sodium hypochlorite prior to inserting into the root canal as they are likely to be contaminated with bacteria.
- The first point (master point) placed in the canal, should fit snugly in the apical part of the root canal to prevent over-extension when compacting further points and to offer some degree of tug-back (resistance to withdrawal) when finger spreaders are removed. The root canal is rarely smooth-sided along its full extent and compaction of gutta percha into irregularities prevents its subsequent withdrawal. The easiest way to achieve this is to choose a gutta percha point slightly larger than the master apical file. After removing any feathered part at its tip with a scalpel, the apical 1–2 mm should be dipped in a suitable solvent such as chloroform for a second and then inserted into the wet root canal to length. It should fit within a millimetre of the end of the root canal preparation. It should then be withdrawn and reinserted several times to prevent it binding in any undercuts. It is often surprising to see what the interior part of the root canal really looks like (Figure 5.30), as the gutta percha will form an accurate impression of the walls of the canal, revealing its anatomy more clearly.

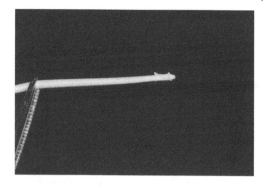

Figure 5.30 Chloroform-customised gutta percha points often reveal the intricate anatomy at the end of the root canal at their tips.

- The canal can be dried and a suitable sealer mixed according to the manufacturer's instructions. If a thin mix is used, when using a sealer such as Roth sealer which uses a powder (mainly zinc oxide) and liquid (eugenol), then it dissolves more easily. It has to be remembered that many cements are thixotropic, i.e. they flow more easily under pressure, therefore a thick mix, which has better properties, can be used.
- The root canal walls are coated with the sealer and the coated master point is inserted to length. A suitably sized finger spreader should be inserted laterally to the master point to create space for a matching accessory point, which can be coated with further sealer at its tip and inserted into the empty space left by the finger spreader. This can be continued until the gutta percha has been firmly compacted in the apical half of the root canal, then a mid-fill radiograph is used to check that the root filling is to length and there are no voids. If everything is fine, then further points can be inserted to complete the obturation.
- A quicker way to fill the root canal is to obturate the apical portion as described above, then searing off all but the compacted apical portion with a Touch 'n Heat unit and applying pressure with a suitable plugger to vertically compact the warmed apical portion. The rest of the root canal can then be filled sequentially, using

thermo-plasticized gutta percha, delivered with a device such as the Obtura® unit. Each addition of gutta percha can be vertically compacted.

Restoration of the access cavity can be completed with a sandwich of IRM® (to provide a bacterial seal), glass ionomer and finally composite. If trauma to the teeth has fractured a greater amount of dentine and enamel, then restoration with a post-retained crown may be necessary. This should be constructed as soon as possible to prevent bacterial leakage and a layer of IRM® used to seal over the remaining few millimetres of gutta percha.

5.6.8.8 Large Apical Foramina

If a tooth has a large apical foramen and a wide root canal, which may have little taper or even a reverse taper, where the root canal at the foramen is wider than the coronal root canal, a different approach needs to be taken. An attempt needs to be made to disinfect the root canal, placing a dressing of calcium hydroxide, then attempting obturation using a material such as MTA. This is compacted into the canal at its apex at a second visit (Figure 5.31a) and sealed with moist, sterile cotton wool under an IRM® filling to allow it to set in a moist environment. Once set after 24 hours, the remaining root canal can be filled with gutta percha (Figure 5.31b).

Prior to the use of MTA, root canals were dressed for a considerable period of time with calcium hydroxide to produce a hard tissue barrier at the end of the tooth, against which thermo-plasticized gutta percha was compacted. This technique is no longer use due to concerns about using long-term dressings of calcium hydroxide, which may cause weakening and fracture of thin-walled teeth.

5.6.8.9 Regeneration

Revascularization of avulsed, incompletely developed teeth with open apices is possible if conditions are favourable, i.e. the tooth is reimplanted quickly and is minimally

(a)   (b)

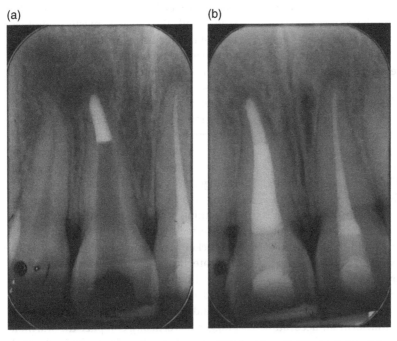

Figure 5.31 An MTA obturation treatment in a tooth with an incompletely formed apex immediately after MTA was placed (a) and following completion of treatment (b).

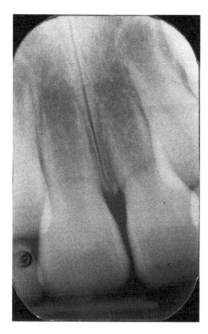

Figure 5.32 A radiograph of traumatised maxillary central incisors in an eight-year-old patient, showing the relatively thin walls of the roots present at this age.

contaminated. More recently, case reports [32,33] have shown that even teeth with necrotic, infected pulps may also undergo revascularization with appropriate treatment. The advantages of this technique are obvious, as immature teeth are difficult to clean with conventional instruments, are difficult to fill due to lack of an apical barrier and their thin walls (Figure 5.32) leave them prone to root fracture.

Initially the technique involved using a triple antibiotic paste (ciprofloxacin, metronidazole, and minocycline) to sterilise the root canal followed by creation of a blood clot in the bacteria-free canal (bleeding from the apical tissues) which allows revascularization to take place. The methods and materials used are evolving and guidelines are now available [34] to help with the management of these teeth.

The terms pulp revascularization or pulp repair have been used to describe this process rather than regeneration, as this latter term implies the pulp is replaced with identical tissues, which has not proven to be the case [35]. Long-term research will discover the degree to which the thickening of a tooth's walls by this method contributes to better survival.

Further details are discussed in Chapter 3 on trauma to juvenile teeth.

5.6.8.10 Surgery

Due to the success of conventional endodontic treatment, surgery is now only needed in those rare instances where conventional treatment has failed or is not possible. Failure is often due to ineffective cleaning of anatomy in the last few millimetres of the root canal, the presence of extra-radicular bacteria surviving on the exterior of the root that are inaccessible to irrigants and due to cyst formation. It can also be used when attempting conventional root canal retreatment may risk the tooth being rendered unrestorable due to the presence of a large post. It is not an alternative to conventional root canal (re)treatment, when this can be completed.

Traumatised teeth do not normally present any particular challenges to surgical treatment. However, the presence of incomplete fractures in the root can be a common finding. Also, surgery completed on teeth where the root canal had become obliterated, prior to developing an infection, present a particular problem. Following exposure of the root tip and removal of granulation tissue, the root tip is apicected, which removes any infected micro-anatomy. Normally, the exposed root filling would be removed to a depth of several millimetres and then filled with MTA. However, in teeth with obliterated canals, resecting the root tip exposes a significant amount of tertiary dentine that may not have been completely disinfected during root canal treatment (Figure 5.32). Therefore, the whole cut surface should be sealed with a dentine-bonded, flowable composite. There is a dedicated material manufactured for this, called Retroplast® (Figures 5.33 and 5.34).

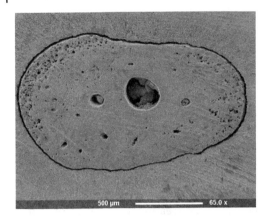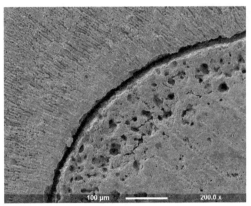

Figure 5.33 A resected root tip of a tooth with an obliterated root canal. Note the porous tertiary dentine in the centre of the tooth formed after dental trauma, which would remain unsealed following preparation and obturation of the main root canal in the centre of the tooth.

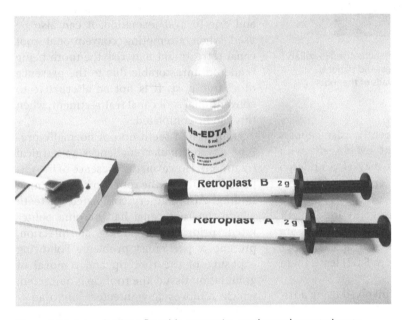

Figure 5.34 Retroplast® is a flowable composite, used to seal resected roots.

5.7 Review

Current recommendations from the International Association for Dental Trauma recommend reviewing teeth after the incident of trauma at one month, three months, six months, and one year, and then yearly afterwards, when clinical and radiographic examination can be repeated. In addition, athletes may need to be examined shortly after their accident for the removal of splints, commencement of root canal treatment, etc. The review times are more frequent initially, as this is when serious complications such as external inflammatory resorption may occur, which needs to be treated quickly to prevent the loss of teeth.

References

1 Glendor, U. (2008). Epidemiology of traumatic dental injuries: a 12-year review of the literature. *Dental Traumatology* 24: 603–611.

2 Karring, T., Nyman, S., Lindhe, J. (1980). Healing following implantation of periodontitis affected roots into bone tissue. *Journal of Clinical Periodontology* 7: 96–105.

3 Nyman, S., Karring, T., Lindhe, J., Plantén, S. (1980). Healing following implantation of periodontitis: affected roots into gingival connective tissue. *Journal of Clinical Periodontology* 7: 394–401.

4 Stålhane, I., Hedegård, B. (1975). Traumatized permanent teeth in children aged 7–15. Part II. *Swedish Dental Journal* 68: 157–169.

5 Ravn, J.J. (1981). Follow-up study of permanent incisors with enamel cracks as a result of an acute trauma. *Scandinavian Journal of Dental Research* 89: 117–123.

6 Robertson, A. (1988). A retrospective analysis of patients with uncomplicated crown fractures and luxation injuries. *Endodontics and Dental Traumatology* 14: 245–256.

7 Ravn, J.J. (1981). Follow-up study of permanent incisors with enamel fractures as a result of an acute trauma *Scandinavian Journal of Dental Research* 89: 213–217.

8 Robertson, A., Andreasen, F.M., Andreasen, J.O., Norén, J.G. (2000). Long-term prognosis of crown-fractured permanent incisors. The effect of stage of root development and associated luxation injury. *International Journal of Paediatric Dentistry* 10: 191–199.

9 Ravn, J.J. (1981). Follow-up study of permanent incisors with enamel-dentin fractures after acute trauma. *Scandinavian Journal of Dental Research* 89: 355–365.

10 Krenkel, C., Grunert, I., Messawarati, S. (1985). Nachuntersuchung von wurzelfrakturierten Zähnen versorgt mit Silcadraht-Klebeschienen. *Zeischrift für Stomatologie* 82: 325–336.

11 Welbury, R.R., Kinirons, M.J., Day, P., Humphreys, K., Gregg, T.A. (2002) Outcomes for root-fractured permanent incisors: a retrospective study. *Pediatric Dentistry* 24: 98–102.

12 Andreasen, F.M., Pedersen B.V. (1985). Prognosis of luxated permanent teeth - the development of pulp necrosis. *Endodontics and Dental Traumatology* 1: 207–220.

13 Kling, M., Cvek, M., Mejare, I. (1986). Rate and predictability of pulp revascularization in therapeutically reimplanted permanent incisors. *Endodontics and Dental Traumatology* 2: 83–89.

14 Miller, S.C. (1950). *Textbook of Periodontia*, 3rd ed. Blakiston, Philadelphia and Toronto.

15 Love, R.M. (1996). Bacterial penetration of the root canal of intact incisor teeth after a simulated traumatic injury. *Dental Traumatology* 12: 289–293.

16 Yanpiset, K., Trope, M. (2000). Pulp revascularization of replanted immature dog teeth after different treatment methods. *Endodontics and Dental Traumatology* 16: 211–217.

17 Andreasen, J.O., Borum, N.K., Jacobsen, H.L., Andreasen, F.M. (1995). Replantation of 400 avulsed permanent incisors. 2. Factors related to pulpal healing. *Endodontics and Dental Traumatology* 11: 59–68.

18 Cvek, M., Cleaton-Jones, P., Austin, J., *et al.* (1990). Effect of topical application of doxycycline on pulp revascularization and periodontal healing in reimplanted monkey incisors. *Dental Traumatology* 6: 170–176.

19 Cvek, M., Cleaton-Jones, P., Austin, J., *et al.* (1990). Pulp revascularization in reimplanted immature monkey incisors: predictability and the effect of antibiotic systemic prophylaxis. *Dental Traumatology* 6: 157–165.

20 Ritter, A.L., Ritter, A.V., Murrah, V., Sigurdsson, A., Trope, M. (2004). Pulp revascularization of replanted immature dog teeth after treatment with minocycline

and doxycycline assessed by laser Doppler flowmetry, radiography, and histology. *Dental Traumatology* 20: 75–84.

21 Tsilingaridis, G., Malmgren, B., Skutberg, C., Malmgren, O. (2015). The effect of topical treatment with doxycycline compared to saline on 66 avulsed permanent teeth: a retrospective case-control study. *Dental Traumatology* 31: 171–176.

22 Andreasen, J.O., Andreasen, F.M., Mejare, I., Cvek, M. (2004). Healing of 400 intra-alveolar root fractures. 2. Effect of treatment factors such as treatment delay, repositioning, splinting type and period and antibiotics. *Dental Traumatology* 20: 203–211.

23 Pitt Ford, T.R., Roberts, G.J. (1991). Immediate and delayed direct pulp capping with the use of a new visible light-cured calcium hydroxide preparation. *Oral Surgery, Oral Medicine, Oral Pathology* 71: 338–342.

24 Cvek, M., Cleaton-Jones, P., Austin, J., Andreasen J,O. (1982). Pulp reactions to exposure after experimental crown fractures or grinding in adult monkeys. *Journal of Endodontics* 9: 391–397.

25 Cvek, M. (1978). A clinical report on partial pulpotomy and capping with calcium hydroxide in permanent incisors with complicated crown fracture. *Journal of Endodontics* 4: 232–237.

26 Bimstein, E., Rotstein, I. (2016). Cvek pulpotomy: revisited. *Dental Traumatology* 32: 438–442.

27 Kakehashi, S., Stanley, H.R., Fitzgerald, W. (1965). The effects of surgical exposures of dental pulpsin germ free and conventional laboratory rats. *Oral Surgery, Oral Medicine, Oral Pathology* 20: 340–349.

28 Ng, Y.L., Mann, V., Gulabivala, K. (2011). A prospective study of the factors affecting outcomes of nonsurgical root canal treatment. Part 1: periapical health. *International Endodontics Journal* 44: 583–609.

29 Setzer, F.C., Shah, S.B., Kohli, M.R., Karabucak, B., Kim, S. (2010). Outcome of endodontic surgery: a meta-analysis of the literature. Part 1: Comparison of traditional root-end surgery and endodontic microsurgery. *Journal of Endodontics* 36:1757–1765.

30 Oginni, A.O., Adekoya-Sofowora, C.A., Kolawole, K.A. (2009). Evaluation of radiographs, clinical signs and symptoms associated with pulp canal obliteration: an aid to treatment decision. *Endodontics and Dental Traumatology* 25: 620–625.

31 Mannan, G., Smallwood, E.R., Gulabivala, K. (2001). Effect of access cavity location and design on degree and distribution of instrumented root canal surface in maxillary anterior teeth. *International Endodontics Journal* 34: 176–183.

32 Iwaya, S., Ikawa, M., Kubota, M. (2001). Revascularization of an immature permanent tooth with apical periodontitis and sinus tract. *Dental Traumatology* 17: 185–187.

33 Banchs, F., Trope, M. (2004). Revascularization of immature permanent teeth with apical periodontitis: new treatment protocol? *Journal of Endodontics* 30: 196–200.

34 Galler, K.M., Krastl, G., Simon, S., *et al.* (2016). European Society of Endodontology position statement: revitalization procedures. *International Endodontics Journal* 49: 717–723.

35 Wang, X., Thibodeau, B., Trope, M., Lin, L.M., Huang, G.T. (2010). Histologic characterization of regenerated tissues in canal space after the revitalization/revascularization procedure of immature dog teeth with apical periodontitis. *Journal of Endodontics* 36 (1): 56–63.

6

Dealing with Tooth Wear in Athletes
Rebecca Moazzez

6.1 Introduction

Tooth wear is a complex process resulting in the loss of tooth tissue. In severe cases, it can affect large surfaces of the tooth, or even a whole tooth. Traditionally tooth wear has been described as four separate processes: attrition, abrasion, erosion, and abfraction [1,2]. Abfraction remains controversial and will not be discussed further in this chapter. One of the difficulties sometimes faced in diagnosis and management of tooth wear is that some wear is natural and occurs as a physiological process associated with age. The difficulty is deciding when the wear is progressing and when treatment may be indicated. Another concept to consider is whether the processes are irreversible or whether early intervention can reverse the process. Whilst historically it was believed that the condition is totally irreversible, this concept is no longer accepted. Whilst the actual loss of tooth substance is irreversible and at present can only be replaced with restorative materials, early stages of demineralisation and initial changes to the tooth surface can be reversed. This results in prevention of loss of tooth tissue and hence preservation of the enamel and dentine. Currently, most of the research and focus is on accurate diagnosis and detection, prevention of further wear and reversal of the processes to try to preserve the natural tooth tissue. Any treatment should be minimally invasive, as far as possible. Although there has been considerable progress in the recent development of biocompatible dental materials and future hope in terms of replacement of tooth tissue with similar substances through stem cell therapy, at present no restorative material has the same favourable properties as natural tooth substance and many years of research are still needed to have an effective stem cell or similar therapy.

6.2 Types of Wear

6.2.1 Attrition

Attrition is the wear of teeth by opposing teeth. Under normal conditions, the teeth only come into contact during mastication and in particular, during swallowing. In patients suffering from bruxism the teeth come into contact at other times during the day or night and generally with increased force. Bruxism can present in the form of clenching or grinding of teeth against each other. Grinding generally occurs at night whilst the patient is asleep, but clenching can happen during the day or at night. In some cases, patients also suffer from temporomandibular (mandibular) dysfunction, which can have a large impact on their quality of life. There are various opinions about the aetiology of bruxism. Occlusal discrepancies, as

Sports Dentistry: Principles and Practice, First Edition. Edited by Peter D. Fine, Chris Louca and Albert Leung.
© 2019 John Wiley & Sons Ltd. Published 2019 by John Wiley & Sons Ltd.
Companion website: www.wiley.com/go/fine/sports_dentistry

well as stress and stress-related medical conditions have been implicated. It is the author's view that in the majority of cases, stress and psychological problems, and conditions such as depression and anxiety are associated with the condition. Although occlusion and occlusal problems are often observed and in most cases need to be addressed in the management of the bruxism, attention to the patient's wellbeing and lifestyle is essential.

6.2.2 Abrasion

Abrasion is wear of teeth by an external object, the most common cause being a toothbrush or other oral hygiene tools. Normal tooth brushing does not generally result in any wear, but excessive amounts of brushing, whether it is the number of times or length of time the brush is in contact with the teeth, excessive force used whilst brushing, and excessive use of an abrasive toothpaste can result in facets of wear representing abrasion.

6.2.3 Dental Erosion

Dental erosion is wear of teeth by acids. The process, including the original source of the acid, is very different to that involved in dental caries (dental decay).

Comparison of the two conditions includes some of the factors below:

- Dental caries is never physiological and therefore the presence of any carious lesion/activity is pathological. This is not the case for dental erosion as a small degree of surface change due to normal consumption of acidic foods and drinks can be considered to be within normal physiological parameters, perhaps even at a microscopic level.
- Dental caries occurs as a result of fermentation of sugary foods and drinks by the bacteria in dental plaque to produce acids, which demineralise the tooth tissue in that area. The process can then progress into further demineralisation, cavitation, and enlargement of the cavity. The source of

acid in dental erosion, however, is either from dietary acidic foods and drinks, or from the stomach, and there are no bacteria involved.

- The main dietary intake affecting initiation and progression of caries is fermented carbohydrates, whereas in the case of erosion it is acidic foods and drinks.
- Surfaces affected by caries are normally covered in plaque, and oral hygiene is generally poor, tooth surfaces affected by erosion are normally clean and plaque-free and are covered by acquired pellicle, which is free from bacteria. In fact, it is unusual to find both conditions in the same patient.
- Dental caries generally affects people from poor socioeconomic background, whereas this is not the case for dental erosion.
- Both conditions are reversible in the initial stages.

6.3   Dental Erosion vs. Erosive Wear

Although the various contributors to tooth wear have been described above and have traditionally been reported as such in the literature, in reality the processes do not occur in isolation. Erosive wear is a relatively new term and represents the interaction between the various processes well [3]. It has recently been defined as a chemical-mechanical process resulting in a cumulative loss of hard dental tissue not caused by bacteria. Figure 6.1 illustrates the interaction of the various concepts. Non- bacterial acids from the diet or regurgitated/vomited from the stomach soften the tooth surface, any subsequent mechanical contact, whether by opposing teeth or through abrasion increases the rate of wear and hence results in tissue loss. The process is dynamic and capable of reversal by biological substances such as saliva and acquired pellicle, or oral hygiene products containing remineralising elements such as fluoride.

This chapter will refer to this condition as 'erosive tooth wear or erosive wear'.

Figure 6.1 Showing the interactions between various factors in erosive wear.

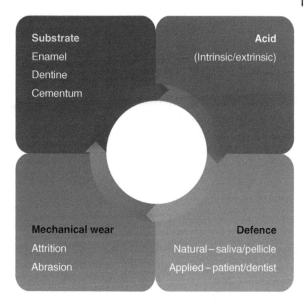

Substrate	Acid
Enamel	(Intrinsic/extrinsic)
Dentine	
Cementum	

Mechanical wear	Defence
Attrition	Natural – saliva/pellicle
Abrasion	Applied – patient/dentist

Erosive wear is caused either by a variety of acidic foods and drinks (dietary erosion) or contact with acidic contents travelling up from the stomach to the mouth. Whilst this represents the two common sources of acids, the process is very complex and a variety of factors influence the initiation and progression of the condition, whilst others help in its prevention and halt its progression. Dietary erosion is also referred to as extrinsic erosion. Other extrinsic causes of dental erosion have been reported in relation to inadequately maintained chlorinated water in swimming pools and occupational hazards such as acidic fumes in car battery factories, but these are now very rare due to tighter regulations.

6.4 Prevalence of Erosive Tooth Wear

Erosive tooth wear is a common condition and there is some evidence suggesting that it is rising. Various studies have suggested that between 3% and 30% of children and adults are affected, with roughly 3% being severely affected. There is a trend for more pronounced rates of wear in younger people. This could be due to increased consumption of acidic foods and drinks and/or lifestyle changes. Although it can be found on any of the teeth, it is more common on the labial and palatal surfaces of the upper anterior teeth and the occlusal surfaces of the molars. The prevalence of gastro-oesophageal reflux disease (GORD), has been reported to be between 4% and 25% of the population. Around 10% of the population seek help for GORD but 'silent reflux', which is GORD without any symptoms is thought to be present is around 25% of the population. The prevalence of erosive wear in those suffering with GORD is said to be between 20% and 30% and GORD is present in around 30% of patients with erosive wear [4–6].

The prevalence is also higher in patients with eating disorders and those with alcohol abuse problems, but more studies are needed to ascertain the real prevalence data.

Erosive wear is a common condition in elite athletes and between 36% to 85% are reported to be affected by the condition. The reasons for this are complicated and can be due to particular nutritional intakes, including but not limited to sports and energy drinks, lifestyle, higher prevalence of eating disorders, and GORD in this group as well as stress-related bruxism.

Although it is very difficult to obtain accurate prevalence data from the literature due to the varied nature of the studies, the groups assessed, and methods of tooth wear assessment, it is clear that erosive wear and the associated medical conditions are prevalent and affect a large population. Moreover, erosive wear is on the increase and therefore detection, diagnosis, and prevention of these conditions is essential.

6.5 Dietary Erosive Wear

Common acidic foods and drinks reported in the literature are: citrus fruit and fruit juices, other fruit juices, carbonated drinks (such as Cola and diet Cola), sports and energy drinks, smoothies, fruit/herbal teas, lemon juice, vinegar and other salad dressings, chewable vitamin C, other acidic medications consumed routinely, and pickles (Table 6.1). Although the pH is a good indicator of the acidity of the food or drink and one of the factors considered most, other factors also need to be taken into account. The titratable acidity, buffering capacity, calcium/phosphate/fluoride content of the drink, and chelation properties should also be considered. Unlike dental caries, there is no critical pH for dissolution of acids and demineralisation can occur at higher pH values if the other factors mentioned above are unfavourable (Table 6.2) [7,8].

The amount and type of acidic food and drink are important factors to consider in

Table 6.1 Examples of erosive foods and drinks.

Citrus fruit
Fresh fruit juices
Diluted squash and other fruit juices
Carbonated drinks
Sports and energy drinks
Smoothies
Herbal teas
Lemon, lemon juice
Vinegar and other acidic salad dressings
Acidic medications such as chewable vitamin C

Table 6.2 Examples of common drinks showing their pH and titratable acidity.

Type of soft drink	pH	Titratable acidity
Coca Cola	2.5	17.5
Sprite	2.5	39
Sprite Zero	3.0	62
Orange juice	3.7	108
Apple juice	3.4	72
Lemon Iced Tea	3.0	24
Redbull	3.3	98
Powerade	3.7	43
Vitamin C (fizzy tablet)	3.9	93

their potential to result in erosive wear. However, other factors such as timing, frequency and method of consumption, mineral content, and temperature of an acidic drink are just as important [9]. The process is further complicated when the nature and dynamics of saliva and pellicle, as well as the soft tissues are also taken into account. Patients who have a habit of swishing and keeping a drink in their mouth are more susceptible to erosive wear. This is due to the fact that fresh acid continues to contact the tooth surface and the contact time between the acid and tooth is prolonged. Consuming acids in between meals as snacks has also been shown to increase the potential for erosive wear. Other factors, such as the temperature of the drink are evident in some herbal teas, which have a higher pH than the more commonly quoted acidic drinks, can result in substantial wear in a short time. The importance of the presence of minerals is evident in that yoghurt, which is acidic, is not an erosive food item due to the high content of calcium and phosphate. Studies have also investigated the effect of addition of calcium and various other minerals to orange juice and various sports drinks, with encouraging outcomes showing a reduction in erosive wear potential. The issue is, however, the negative effect on the taste of the drinks and acceptability to the consumers.

A variety of medical conditions are also connected to erosive wear:

- Gastro-oesophageal reflux disease (GORD)
- Laryngopharyngeal reflux (LPR)
- Eating disorders (anorexia and bulimia nervosa)
- Conditions resulting in reduced salivary flow such as Sjogren's syndrome
- Medications resulting in reduced salivary flow
- Medical conditions and pregnancy resulting in chronic vomiting
- Rumination, in particular in patients with learning disabilities
- Chronic alcoholism.

6.6 Gastro-Oesophageal Reflux Disease (GORD)/ Laryngopharyngeal Reflux (LPR)

GORD is a condition where the contents of the stomach are regurgitated back through the lower oesophageal sphincter (LOS), up to the oesophagus. In some cases the stomach contents travel up the oesophagus further, past the upper oesophageal sphincter (UOS), and reach the pharynx/larynx and finally the oral cavity. Small amounts of regurgitation into the oesophagus is normal; however, in patients suffering with GORD, the amounts are excessive and result in pathological reflux. In most cases the cause is transient relaxations of the LOS, an incompetent LOS, or disorders of the muscular function of the oesophagus. Gastroenterologists often refer to the Montreal definition of GORD, which is, 'A condition which develops when the reflux of stomach contents causes troublesome symptoms and/or complications. It is normally classified as: ≥2 heartburn episodes/ week and adversely affecting an individual's wellbeing [10,11].

Generally an area 5 cm above the LOS is the position for assessment of the presence of the refluxate; however, in some patients it can travel further up. When it travels passed the UOS and into the pharynx the term LPR is sometimes used. In most cases the refluxate is acidic, although it can occasionally be non-acidic or gaseous.

The presence of LPR and an acidic refluxate are more likely to result in erosive wear as there is more likelihood of the acidic contents reaching the oral cavity and coming into contact with the teeth.

Symptoms of reflux are many and varied, but the two most common symptoms of GORD are: heartburn and regurgitation. Table 6.3 contains a more comprehensive list of the symptoms and Table 6.4 compares GORD and LPR. Dysphagia is a difficulty in swallowing, globus is a feeling of a lump in the throat, and hoarseness is a change in the voice (Table 6.3). Barratt's oesophagus refers to a change in the lining of the oesophagus and can be pre-malignant. It is caused as a result of repeated insult to the lining of the oesophagus by the refluxate. Although the prevalence of Barratt's oesophagus is low, the potential to result in adenocarcinoma of the oesophagus indicates the need for correct diagnosis and control of the acid in GORD. In some cases, GORD is 'silent', in other words there are no symptoms and the only sign is erosive tooth wear. This does

Table 6.3 Symptoms of GORD.

Oesophageal/typical symptoms	Extra-oesophageal/ atypical symptoms
Heartburn	Cardiac: non-cardiac chest pain
Regurgitation	Pulmonary: chronic cough, asthma
Belching	ENT: hoarseness, globus, pharyngitis, laryngitis
Bloating	Dental: Erosive wear
Dysphagia	
Nausea	
Barratt's oesophagus	
Adenocarcinoma	

Table 6.4 Comparison between GORD and LPR.

Symptoms	GORD	LPR
Heartburn and/or regurgitation	++++	+
Hoarseness, cough, dysphagia, globus	+	++++
Test results		
Abnormal oesophageal pH monitoring	++++	++
Abnormal pharyngeal pH monitoring	+	++++
Response to Treatment		
Effectiveness of dietary and lifestyle modifications	+	+
Successful treatment with single-dose PPIs	+++	++
Successful treatment with twice-daily PPIs	+++	++++

raise the point about the importance of detection and diagnosis of erosive wear and the identification of the source of acid by dental professionals [12].

Traditionally GORD was diagnosed by endoscopy, followed by manometry (assessing the motility of the oesophagus and determining the position of the LOS), followed by 24-hour pH measurement. The results were then analysed and a diagnosis of GORD was determined. The 24-hour test was the gold standard. There are problems with this method in that it is not designed to detect non-acidic or gaseous reflux. Moreover, it is very uncomfortable as the pH catheter is passed through the nose down to 5 cm above the LOS and remains there for 24 hours, whilst the patient is asked to carry on with 'normal life'. 24 hours may also not be long enough, as some patients experience reflux episodes less frequently. The position of 5 cm above the LOS is useful for detection of refluxate that stays lower down in the oesophagus, but is unable to detect high reflux and LPR. New methods of detection and diagnosis include the use of impedance, along with pH, to detect all types of reflux (acidic, non-acidic, gaseous), multiple pH catheters to measure reflux higher up the oesophagus and in the pharynx, and a new wireless system (the Bravo capsule), implanted to the mucosa of the oesophagus during endoscopy, which can measure pH for up to 96 hours and is comfortable, as there are no wires attached. These are some of the modern improvements in the diagnosis of the conditions.

In terms of management of GORD, the main route is the use of medication alongside lifestyle modifications. The main medication, which is highly effective is proton pump inhibitors (PPIs). PPIs work well in controlling the acid and improving the symptoms dramatically, but, like most medications, have side effects such as GI infections and hip fractures. There is also the problem of a rebound effect when the patient stops taking the medication, where excessive acid production can result after prolonged suppression, resulting in such severe symptoms that drive the patient back to taking the medication.

6.7 Eating Disorders

Eating disorders are generally divided into anorexia nervosa (AN), bulimia nervosa (BN), and other groups that do not fully fall into a clear category of AN or BN and have features of both.

AN generally affects between 0.2% to 2% of the population and BN has been reported to affect between 1% and 3%. The prevalence is much higher in females with a tenfold increase in risk. Both conditions tend to be common in highly intelligent middle- and upper-class societies, AN affecting a slightly younger age range (prevalent in teenagers) and BN in a slightly older age group (majority females in the 20s). The prevalence of eating disorders has been reported to be higher in elite athletes and higher in women than men in this group. Anorexics have a restricted diet and will only eat 'safe', non-calorific foods and drinks, which include fruit, vegetables, and diet drinks, while bulimics tend to have binging episodes when they consume large amounts of food and drink, and this is followed by vomiting (the binge/purge cycle). Some anorexics also have vomiting episodes. What makes this even more complicated is the positive correlation between AN and BN, and GORD, reduced salivary flow rate and buffering capacity, and hence dry mouth and changes in the electrolyte balance in this group of people. Eating disorders are related to perceptions of body image and dieting, but there is a strong psychological element of control of body image and often depression that accompanies the obsession with losing weight. Sports that encourage leanness have been reported to have a higher prevalence of females suffering from AN.

A correlation between eating disorders and erosive wear has been reported. This occurs in both those suffering from AN and BN. Although those with a habit of vomiting have a higher risk of severe erosion (present in BN sufferers but also in some AN sufferers), anorexics who do not vomit also suffer from condition due to restrictive acidic diets, GORD and dry mouth.

6.8 Effects of Alcohol

Frequent consumption of alcohol can result in erosive wear in two ways: the acidic nature of the alcoholic drink or the resulting vomiting and reflux/regurgitation. Professional wine tasters' teeth have frequent exposure to acidic wines and therefore suffer from dietary erosive wear.

6.9 Rumination

Rumination is a fairly uncommon condition affecting mainly people with learning disabilities, but has also been reported in highly intelligent individuals and professionals. It occurs as a result of voluntary regurgitation of solid and liquid foods from the stomach back into the mouth, rechewing and swallowing again. The psychological nature of the

condition is not well understood, and there may be an association with GORD and resulting incompetence of the LOS. Individuals suffering from this condition are generally embarrassed by it and hence unlikely to disclose the habit, which makes diagnosis challenging. Rumination can result in severe erosive wear, as regurgitated food from the stomach is highly acidic and erosive.

6.10 Short-term Causes of Erosive Wear

Pregnant women often complain of sickness, and some suffer from frequent episodes of vomiting, in particular in the first trimester. Erosive wear has been reported in pregnancy as a result, although the condition is self-limiting and once the vomiting stops, no further erosive wear occurs. However, it is important to bear this in mind and put in place preventive measures to avoid excessive wear of teeth during this period.

Consumption of acidic medications have also been reported as a cause of erosive wear, examples include soluble vitamin C and asthma inhalers. There is some debate as to whether the inhalers are acidic or it is the resultant relaxation of the LOS that causes regurgitation and erosive wear.

6.11 The Role of Saliva and Pellicle in Erosive Wear

Saliva and pellicle provide natural defence mechanisms against erosive wear. This protection is effective prior to, during, and after an erosive challenge. Saliva helps in removal, buffering, and neutralisation of acids, and acts as a reservoir for minerals such as calcium, phosphorus, and fluoride. Conflicting reports have been given in the literature regarding the role of saliva in erosive wear, but recent research strongly supports the positive protective effect of saliva against erosive wear. Acids entering the oral cavity and hence contacting the tooth surface are cleared within a few minutes. The importance of this has been demonstrated by investigating the prevalence of erosive wear in patients who suffer from dry mouth. Patients with Sjogrens disease, for example, have a higher prevalence of erosive wear and GORD than those with normal salivary flow. Physically active young adults have also been shown to have reduced salivary flow compared with a matched age group who do not take part in sports.

Pellicle has a crucial role in protection against erosive wear, forming immediately after brushing and directly contacting the tooth surface. Pellicle in effect forms a diffusible barrier between the tooth and the oral cavity. Using recent methods such as proteomics (large-scale experimental analysis of proteins), it has been shown to contain over 130 different proteins. Calcium-binding proteins such as Statherin have been shown to be present in smaller amounts in patients with erosive wear, proteins such as mucins can have a protective lubricating effects, and others such as carbonic anhydrase have a role in neutralisation of acids. The combination of the proteins and the minerals present in pellicle offer protection by the above mechanisms, as well as the provision of a reservoir of minerals next to the tooth. The protective effects of pellicle, however, can be overcome with repeated and severe acid challenges [13–16].

6.12 Distribution of Wear Facets and Colour as an Indication of Progression

Erosive wear can theoretically affect all surfaces of all teeth and in very severe cases this does happen, with the crowns of teeth wearing down to the roots. However, typically the most commonly affected teeth are the upper anterior teeth and the molars. Dietary erosive wear affects the labial surfaces of the upper anterior teeth and regurgitation erosion affects the palatal surfaces of the upper anterior teeth and the occlusal surfaces of the molars. This is, however, dependent on the

method of drinking and the dynamics within the oral cavity, which are dependent on the flow of saliva and movement of the soft tissues, as well as the direction in which the refluxate travels. As an example, some patients with nocturnal reflux only have wear of their teeth on one side as they have a preferred side for sleeping (Figures 6.2–6.5).

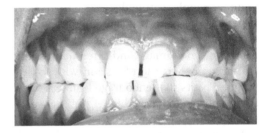

Figure 6.2 Picture showing erosive wear of teeth due to nocturnal reflux. The teeth on the left side are more affected than the right.

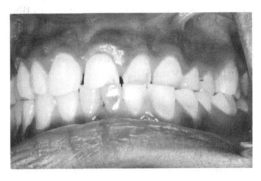

Figure 6.3 Picture showing erosive wear of teeth due to nocturnal reflux. The teeth on the left side are more affected than the right. This picture shows the wear facets more clearly on the left side.

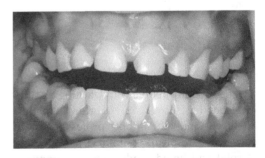

Figure 6.4 Labial surfaces of upper and lower anterior teeth affected by wear. Early erosive wear is evident on the LL 1 and LL2. The upper teeth have been covered with composite as a temporary measure.

The colour of the lesion can provide some indication of the activity of the erosion. Wear facets that are not stained are usually indicative of active wear, whereas stained facets represent wear that may be stable (Figures 6.7 and 6.8).

The shape of the wear could indicate whether a lesion is, for example, primarily due to abrasion (Figure 6.6a) or erosion (Figure 6.6b).

The case of GORD in Figure 6.7 is not progressing and is stable. The patient is on PPIs for the treatment of GORD and control of acids, which in turn has resulted in the stability of the erosive wear.

A relatively recent scoring system: The Basic Erosive Wear Examination (BEWE) is a very useful tool for a quick assessment of the presence and severity of wear. BEWE uses a four-point scale (0–3) for each sextant, with 0 representing no wear and 3 representing severe wear affecting more than 50% of the surface (Table 6.5) [17].

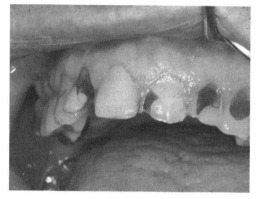

Figure 6.7 Labial stained wear facets in a patient that has had erosive wear as a result of GORD.

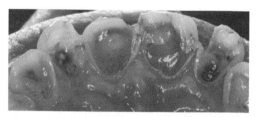

Figure 6.8 Palatal surfaces of the teeth affected by erosive wear due to GORD.

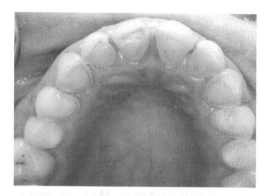

Figure 6.5 Palatal surfaces of the upper anterior teeth affected by erosive wear.

(a) (b)

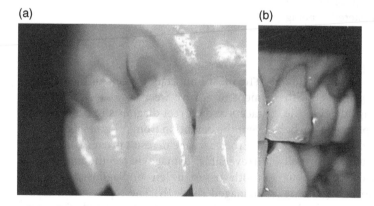

Figure 6.6 (a) A wedge-shaped wear facet on the labial surface of a canine tooth primarily due to abrasion. (b) Wear facets on the labial/buccal surfaces of the teeth primarily due to erosion, having a typical washed out/dish-shaped appearance.

Table 6.5 BEWE index for scoring erosive wear.

Score	Criteria
0	No erosive tooth wear
1	Initial loss of surface texture
2	Hard tissue loss less than 50% of the surface area
3	Hard tissue loss greater than 50% of the surface area

One of the main areas for future research is detection of early erosion and demineralisation in vivo. At present, the initial surface changes need to be detected visually, which normally results in loss of surface characteristics of the enamel, the presence of grooves, and loss of the shine of the enamel. As the process continues, the result is further visible tissue loss.

6.13 Erosive Wear in Elite Athletes

Erosive wear is prevalent in elite athletes and been reported to be between 36% and 85%. Poor oral health, including erosive wear, adversely affects the quality of life and performance of athletes. There are many reasons for this, including pain, sensitivity, and difficulty eating, as well as appearance. Many reports have linked this to the consumption of sports/energy drinks. Energy drinks and various other products are marketed as being advantageous over water for hydration and improving performance. There is a no doubt that the sports drinks industry is very lucrative and a multi-million or billion pound entity. It is a rapidly growing market with new 'enhanced' products being added to the market. Many claim these products to be superior for hydration and are advertised to increase strength, power, speed, and overall performance. There is also a debate about the need for hydration prior to feeling thirsty and prior to commencing exercise, and using a drink that contains additional elements such as electrolytes, carbohydrates, proteins, acids, and other ingredients, such as acids, rather than water. The opposite view is that the danger of dehydration in a healthy athlete is less than that of over-hydration.

Performance is the centre of an elite athlete's professional life and anything that could it would be welcome. It is therefore difficult to suggest completely avoiding these products on the basis of improved oral health. On the other hand, although there have been some studies on the adverse effects of these products and their erosive nature, most of these have been carried out in the laboratory, without taking into consideration the effects of saliva and the complicated processes involved in erosive wear in vivo. There is also no evidence to date that links sports drinks to poor oral health and erosive wear in this group. It is vital to ascertain the aetiology of this erosive wear, in order to devise an appropriate preventive plan. However, one needs to have a more holistic approach and consider the overall nutrition plan and dietary intake, and the possible role of GORD, eating disorders, and reduced salivary flow, as well as simply targeting sports drinks. Certain groups of athletes are at particular risk of erosive wear, including those involved in endurance training, in particular female runners and also swimmers. More research is needed to understand the complicated interactions that result in a higher susceptibility in some groups [18–22].

6.14 Management of Erosive Wear

The most important aspects of the management of erosive wear are detection of wear facets and correct diagnosis in order to prevent the condition from progressing.

Erosive wear can result in catastrophic and irreversible damage to teeth and loss of tooth tissue if left undiagnosed and not managed correctly. The replacement of the lost tooth tissue is complicated, time-consuming, and expensive, involving full-mouth rehabilitation in severe cases. Although many biocompatible dental materials are available and recent developments have resulted in very favourable restorative materials, none of the materials match the favourable properties of enamel or dentine, and therefore preservation of the natural tooth tissues should be the ultimate goal.

The following steps are recommended for the management of erosive wear, although, depending on the extent of wear, patient's wishes, and other circumstances, the order may have to be adjusted:

1) Correct diagnosis and detection of the wear facets
2) Preventive program
3) Monitoring
4) Reassessment
5) Minimally invasive treatment
6) Comprehensive treatment including full mouth rehabilitation
7) Maintenance.

The aims are to:

1) Reduce and possibly eliminate the sources of acids
2) Neutralise the acids
3) Strengthen defence mechanisms
4) Protect tooth surfaces
5) Strengthen the tooth tissue.

6.14.1 Diagnosis and Detection

Diagnosis of erosive wear requires the usual steps in diagnosis of any condition, which include a thorough history, detailed extra-oral and intra-oral examinations, as well as any necessary special tests. A thorough history of the patient's perception of the wear is essential. Some patients present with complaints regarding the appearance of the teeth, sensitivity or pain, and problems eating and chewing, whereas other have no specific complaints and the condition is detected and diagnosed by a dental professional.

The history should include assessment of any symptoms associated with the teeth, a comprehensive dietary history, which should include a diet diary recording at least four days (two weekdays and two weekend days), assessment of symptoms and signs of GORD/LPR, and assessment of any signs and symptoms of mandibular dysfunction and bruxism. A detailed medical history is needed to investigate any medical conditions that could be relevant, as detailed above, as well as alcohol intake and pregnancy. Oral hygiene habits need to be assessed in detail, including the type of toothbrush and toothpaste used, inter-proximal methods of cleaning, use of mouth washes as well as duration, and force and frequency of brushing. Any habits need to be discussed, such as the method of consumption of drinks and pen chewing.

Table 6.6 contains a list of various aspects of the diet history.

It is also important to ask questions about the patient's lifestyle. Some of these are centred on family life, occupation, and general work/life balance. The important relevant points are frequency and timings of consumption of food and drink, snacking, and eating late at night. Others include stress and recent stressful life events, activities and sports, and any habits related to sport activities such as consumption of sports drinks.

Additional records, questionnaires, and special tests include: photographs, diet diary (longer period), reflux symptoms questionnaire, questions regarding a possible eating disorder, dated study models, and necessary radiographs. There are various validated reflux disease symptoms questionnaires that have a fairly robust specificity and sensitivity,

Table 6.6 Factors to consider when assessing acidic dietary intake

Amount
Type
Frequency
Timing in relation to meals
Method of consumption
Timing of tooth brushing and other habits
Consumption of foods and drinks with potential for neutralisation afterwards

and would be a very good tool for practitioners to use as a guide to possible GORD being the source of acid in undiagnosed patients. One such example is a 12-item self-administered questionnaire assessing the frequency and severity of heartburn, regurgitation (the two most typical symptoms of GORD), and a few other symptoms. These questionnaires have been shown to be reliable in the primary care setting for assistance in diagnosis, as well as monitoring the effect of treatment on the symptoms. This could be a very useful, minimally invasive tool for dental professionals in cases where a referral for diagnosis using invasive methods is not indicated or not accepted by the patient.

6.14.2 Preventive Programme

6.14.2.1 Reduction of Aetiological Factors, Neutralisation of Acids and Strengthening the Defence Mechanisms

Once a correct diagnosis is made and the source of acids and possible other factors such as attrition and abrasion have been ascertained, the main aim is to eliminate as many of these factors as possible. It is of course not always easy to identify and eliminate all of the sources at the first attempt and the process needs to be continued.

Changing behaviours is challenging and it is vital that any advice on lifestyle and dietary changes are tailored to the patient and not given as a generalised preventive advice. There is some evidence to suggest eating acidic foods and drinks in between meals is associated with erosion. There is also evidence that the method of drinking and eating, and the contact time between the acids and the teeth has a large influence. Brushing after consumption of acids has been debated and at present the jury is out. However, until more evidence is available, the advice should be to brush teeth before consuming acids or delay brushing.

Dietary advice should:

1) Be assessed comprehensively using a diet diary
2) Be tailored to each patient

3) Include not only the amount of acid intake, but also timing, frequency, and method of intake. The aim should be to limit acidic intake to mealtimes, reducing the frequency and ensuring contact time with the teeth is minimal by avoiding swishing the drink in the mouth (Table 6.6)
4) Include discussions on what foods and drinks can replace the acidic items
5) Include assessment and advice regarding refluxogenic foods and drinks (as well as acidic intake) in patients suffering with or suspected to suffer with GORD. Some of these foods are: fatty foods, onions, citrus fruit, spicy food, tomatoes, and coffee. Advice should also be given regarding avoiding large meals and eating late at night.

Other advice regarding lifestyle changes for GORD patients includes: using pillows to be upright in bed, not eating prior to exercise, smoking cessation, reduction of alcohol intake, stress management, and weight loss.

Neutralisation of acids can be targeted by drinking water after consumption of acids, eating a piece of cheese or chewing sugar-free chewing gum. Chewing gum can be effective in neutralising acids in the mouth as well as regurgitated acids in the oesophagus in cases of GORD [24,25].

Various fluoride-containing products are available for use to help in the defence against erosive wear. Although more specific research is needed, there is general consensus that fluoride products are effective in the prevention of demineralisation rather than induction of remineralisation. Toothpastes containing sodium fluoride have some effect in mild erosive wear, but those containing stannous fluoride, as well as toothpastes with higher concentration of fluoride (5000 ppm) have been shown to be more effective. There is also some evidence suggesting the use of a fluoride-containing mouth rinses, as well as toothpastes, and application of high-fluoride varnish at regular intervals can be beneficial [26,27].

Other products have also been investigated for protection against erosive wear. One example is casein phosphopeptide amorphous calcium phosphate (CCP-ACP), which is commercially available as tooth mousse. Tooth mousse has been shown to be effective by allowing a mineral precipitate to form on the surface of the enamel. Another more recent concept is the use of protease inhibitors to preserve the collagen matrix in dentine. A commonly used product that is a protease inhibitor, chlorhexidine, has shown some promising results in protection of dentine against progression of erosive wear.

Natural defence mechanisms including saliva and pellicle play a major role in protection of teeth against erosive wear. Efforts should be made to improve the protective effects of saliva and pellicle in patients at risk of erosive wear. Some methods, such as chewing sugar-free and non-acidic chewing gum have already been mentioned, but other developments are the addition of substances such as casein, mucins, and lipids to products to enhance the protective effect of the pellicle. In future, salivary and pellicle markers can be utilised to identify patients at risk, which helps in ensuring prevention is planned early in the process. An example is the presence of pepsin in saliva, indicating susceptibility to GORD-related erosive wear.

In patients where attrition due to bruxism is suspected, provision of a mouth guard is indicated. There are several types available, but the author's preference is a full coverage upper hard acrylic splint ('Michigan' splint) in most cases. Soft splints are useful as a temporary measure to overcome symptoms of TMJ dysfunction. Simultaneous efforts to manage stress should also be advised. Various stress management strategies, including exercise, yoga, acupuncture, and hypnosis are available, but these are all a matter of personal choice by the patient. In some cases, appropriate referrals for psychological assessment and psychotherapy are indicated, and some patients need medications such as antidepressants to help improve the symptoms. Occlusal analysis and, in a minority of cases, simple occlusal adjustment may be needed.

6.14.2.2 Protection of the Surface and Strengthening the Tooth Tissue

Protection of the tooth surface can be carried out by a variety of methods. High-fluoride varnishes have been shown to protect the tooth against erosive wear if applied on a regular basis by a dental professional. Dentine bonding agents (DBAs) have also been shown to have a protective effect that tends to last around three months. Fissure sealants seem to last slightly longer than DBAs, perhaps up to around six months. Composite restorations of wear facets that have a typical dish-shaped appearance, resulting in wear of dentine, and leaving a rim of unsupported enamel behind, could also be viewed as protection. If this procedure is not carried out, the unsupported enamel is likely to fracture, resulting in further loss of tooth structure [28,29].

6.14.3 Monitoring

Monitoring of erosive wear is essential and must continue until such time as the wear has ceased. This usually means monitoring of mild wear, while diagnosing the aetiological factors and planning a preventive program. Monitoring of moderate to severe wear prior to or during any active treatment is needed until such time that a diagnosis has been reached, all aetiological factors have been removed, and the wear is stable over a period of time. If this is not carried out, there is no objective way of knowing if the wear is progressing or at what rate. Embarking on complicated treatment without this period of monitoring could result in failure if the wear is progressing, as the tooth tissue will continue to wear around the new restorations. Monitoring the progress of wear can also help determine the correct timing of any treatment that may be indicated.

At the present time the most commonly used method of monitoring is with dated study models. This method is easy and cheap, but has the disadvantage of the need for visible changes to the surface before any change can be detected. The progress of wear is generally slow and therefore study models need to be rechecked no sooner than six months to one year in most cases. Other useful indicators are existing restorations as reference points to any wear of the teeth occurring surrounding them, as well as the colour of the wear facets. Stained wear facets are more likely to be inactive than fresh, clean-looking enamel and dentine. In future there may be possibilities of monitoring more accurately using intra-oral scanners.

6.14.4   Treatment

Active treatment and restoration of teeth affected by erosive wear should only be carried out if there is a good indication, and as far as possible be minimally invasive and conservative. The difficulty in most cases is lack of adequate tooth tissue, resulting in short clinical crowns and lack of adequate tooth structure. Another difficulty often encountered is lack of inter-occlusal space due to the slow nature of the progress of erosive tooth wear, resulting in dentoalveolar compensation. It is very unusual for restorations to be carried out in a conformative occlusal scheme as a result. In most cases the occlusal scheme will need to be reorganised. In cases of localised tooth wear this is with the use of the Dahl principle and in more generalised cases a complete occlusal rehabilitation may be necessary. In some cases this may need to be accompanied by crown lengthening procedures to improve the clinical crown heights for increased retention of restorations.

Some indications for treatment can be listed as follows:

1) Patient's wishes
2) Appearance
3) Unsupported enamel and chipping of incisal edges
4) Sensitivity or pain
5) Short clinical crown
6) Excessive loss of tooth tissue making future treatment difficult
7) Changes in occlusion including vertical dimensions.

6.14.4.1   Materials of Choice

Direct and indirect restorations can be used to restore teeth affected by erosive wear. The most appropriate material for direct restorations is composite resin. In recent years, developments in composite materials in terms of bonding to tooth tissue, appearance, and various other improvements in polishability and reduction in shrinkage have resulted in excellent materials. Bonding to enamel and dentine can be carried out with the available DBAs (dentine bonding agents). Glass ionomers are not as commonly used in case the sources of acids have not been fully eliminated, which could result in rapid wear of the restorations. Bonded composite restorations have the advantage of good appearance, adhesion, and better retention, as well as strengthening the remaining tooth structure. They are also very conservative, as in most cases there is no or little preparation of the tooth required.

Indirect restorations include labial/buccal and palatal veneers, cuspal coverage inlays/onlays and crowns. Composite or porcelain veneers can be used. The decision depends on a variety of factors, such as susceptibility to staining, which affects composite resin and not porcelain (smoking, coffee, and red wine are examples), the need to remove some tooth tissue for porcelain veneers (this is generally not indicated for composite resin), occlusion, shade matching, etc. On the whole the author's preference in most cases is for composite, due to the conservative nature of the material as well as the ease of repair and adjustments. The appearance of these veneers using modern materials closely matches porcelain. As far as restoration of posterior teeth is concerned, gold, composite, or porcelain can be used, depending on the patient's preferences with regards to the appearance (gold still being a conservative material with good long-term outcomes if accepted by the patient), as well as other considerations such as remaining tooth structure and occlusion.

There is a continuing debate regarding the advantages and disadvantages of composite restorations compared with crowns. Composite resin restorations are more conservative of natural tooth tissue, have a good appearance and can be repaired and adjusted easily. They do, however, need maintenance more regularly and require the patient to commit to this maintenance program. Crowns, on the other hand, generally last longer without any need for maintenance, but are much more destructive of tooth tissue, and failure of crowns is generally more complicated. Crowning teeth could result in loss of vitality of the tooth, hence requiring root canal treatment, and loss of retention or fracture of the tooth. Both treatment modalities are of course needed, but it is the author's preference to keep the treatment as conservative as possible, only using indirect restorations that need removal of tooth tissue in teeth that have already lost a substantial amount of tissue to a minimum and when absolutely necessary.

6.14.4.2 Localised Wear

In cases where the wear facets are localised and not in contact with opposing teeth (such as labial surfaces of the upper anterior teeth or bucco-cervical lesions), a conformative approach can be chosen. These facets can be restored with direct composite restorations. When wear affects the palatal surfaces of the upper anterior teeth or occlusal surfaces of the posterior teeth together with dento-alveolar compensation, the Dahl principle is generally used [30,31].

Space is generally created by one of the following methods:

1) Dahl appliance – metal (removable or fixed) (Figure 6.11)
2) Dahl appliance – composite (direct or indirect) (Figures 6.9 and 6.10)
3) Leaving temporaries/provisionals 'high'

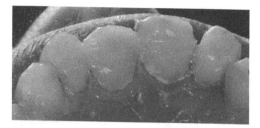

Figure 6.9 Palatal restorations of the teeth shown in Figure 6.8 with Dahl effect composite restorations.

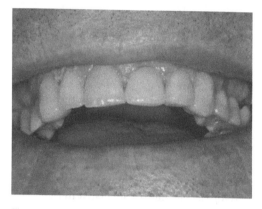

Figure 6.10 Labial surfaces of the teeth shown in Figure 6.7 showing indirect composite restorations.

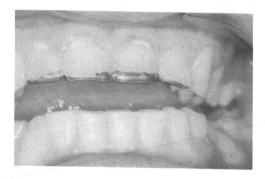

Figure 6.11 A fixed metal Dahl appliance.

4) Leaving definitive crowns 'high'
5) Orthodontics (anterior bite plane or fixed appliances)
6) Occlusal adjustment.

These appliances have not been used frequently in recent years and have been replaced mainly with composite resin.

6.14.4.3 Generalised Wear

In cases of generalised wear, most if not all of the teeth affected by wear will need to be treated. This is often in the form of full-mouth rehabilitation. The steps for success of this treatment are complicated and planning of the case for a successful outcome is essential. Planning involves the use of articulated study models in retruded contact position (RCP), photographs, diagnostic wax-ups, and intra-oral mock-ups. In cases where crowns are to be used, it is generally advised to carry out composite restorations initially and copy the occlusal scheme to construct provisional restorations. Once the provisional restorations have been in place for a reasonable length of time and are successful, the occlusal scheme can then be transferred to final restorations. The occlusal scheme generally involves restorations being made in RCP and at increased overall vertical dimension (OVD). Full-mouth rehabilitation of erosive wear cases is generally complicated, therefore a referral to a specialist in this field is recommended.

In cases of both localised and generalised wear, treatment may also include crown lengthening procedures to improve the clinical crown height.

6.14.4.4 Maintenance

On completion of treatment, and in particular in cases where the aetiology indicated an element of attrition caused by bruxism, it is advisable to provide the patient with a mouth guard to protect the restorations.

The patient should then be placed on a maintenance programme which includes:

1) Regular assessment
2) Continuation of preventive program
3) Monitoring
4) Repair of restorations when needed.

6.14.5 Multi-disciplinary Approach

Erosive wear as described above has various aetiological factors, some relating to nutritional habits, lifestyle choices, life events, and susceptibility, as well as medical conditions. The condition in elite athletes is even more complicated by various nutritional and training routines, and habits related to the various sports, as well as possible dehydration and the need for rehydration and energy supplements.

A multi-disciplinary understanding and awareness of the signs and symptoms, as well as other factors that are related to the condition is the gold standard. This can result in appropriate and timely referrals for diagnosis and management.

Management is also best carried out by a multi-disciplinary team which can include: general dental practitioners and other dental health professionals, general medical practitioners, specialists, gastroenterologists, nutritionists, and psychiatrists/psychologists.

References

1 Addy, M., Shellis, R.P. (2006). Interaction between attrition, abrasion and erosion in tooth wear. *Monographs in Oral Science* 20: 17–31.

2 Amaechi, B.T., Higham, S.M., Edgar, W.M. (2003). Influence of abrasion in clinical manifestation of human dental erosion. *Journal of Oral Rehabilitation* 30: 407–413.

3 Carvalho, T.S., Colon, P., Ganss, C., et al. (2016). Consensus Report of the European Federation of Conservative Dentistry: erosive tooth wear diagnosis and management. *Swiss Dental Journal* 126: 342–346.

4 Jaeggi, T., Lussi, A. (2014). Prevalence, incidence and distribution of erosion. In: *Erosive Tooth Wear* (ed. Lussi, A., Ganss, C.) Vol. 25. Karger, Basel: 55–74.

5 Bartlett, D.W., Lussi, A., West, N.X., et al. (2013). Prevalence of tooth wear on buccal and lingual surfaces and possible risk factors in young European adults. *Journal of Dentistry* 41: 1007–1013.

6 Järvinen, V.K., Rytömaa, I.I., Heinonen, O.P. (1991). Risk factors in dental erosion. *Journal of Dental Research* 70: 942–947.

7 Lussi, A., Jaeggi, T., Zero, D. (2004). The role of diet in the aetiology of dental erosion. *Caries Research* 38(Suppl 1): 34–44.

8 Milosevic, A. (2010). Dental erosion in a series of referred patients was statistically associated with gastric reflux, acidic drink intake of more than 0.5 L per day, and low salivary buffering capacity. *Journal of Evidence Based Dental Practice* 10: 176–178.

9 Moazzez, R., Smith, B.G., Bartlett, D.W. (2000). Oral pH and drinking habit during ingestion of a carbonated drink in a group of adolescents with dental erosion. *Journal of Dentistry* 28: 395–397.

10 Dent, J., El-Serag, H.B., Wallander, M.A., Johansson, S. (2005). Epidemiology of gastro-oesophageal reflux disease: a systematic review. *Gut* 54: 710–717.

11 Fox, M., Forgacs, I. (2006). Gastro-oesophageal reflux disease. *British Medical Journal* 332: 88–93.

12 Moazzez, R., Bartlett, D, Anggiansah, A. (2004). Dental erosion, gastro-oesophageal reflux disease and saliva: how are they related? *Journal of Dentistry* 32: 489–494.

13 Bartlett, D.W., Ganss, C., Lussi, A. (2008). Basic Erosive Wear Examination (BEWE): a new scoring system for scientific and clinical needs. *Clinical Oral Investigations* 12(Suppl 1): S65–S68.

14 Hara, A.T., Zero, D.T. (2014). The potential of saliva in protecting against dental erosion. *Monographs in Oral Science* 25: 197–205.

15 Zwier, N., Huysmans, M.C., Jager D.H., et al. (2013). Saliva parameters and erosive wear in adolescents. *Caries Research* 47: 548–552.

16 Hannig, M., Hannig, C. (2014). The pellicle and erosion. *Monographs in Oral Science* 25: 206–214.

17 Carpenter, G. Cotroneo, E., Moazzez, R., et al. Composition of enamel pellicle from dental erosion patients. *Caries Research* 48: 361–367.

18 Moazzez, R., Bartlett, D., Anggiansah, A. (2005). The effect of chewing sugar-free gum on gastro-esophageal reflux. *Journal of Dental Research* 84: 1062–1065.

19 Smoak, B.R., Koufman, J.A. (2001). Effects of gum chewing on pharyngeal and esophageal pH. *Annals of Otology, Rhinology and Laryngology* 110: 1117–1119.

20 O'Toole, S., Bartlett, D.W., Moazzez, R. (2016). Efficacy of sodium and stannous fluoride mouthrinses when used before single and multiple erosive challenges. *Australian Dental Journal* 61: 10.1111/adj.12418.

21 O'Toole, S., Mistry, M., Mutahar, M., Moazzez, R., Bartlett, D. (2015). Sequence of stannous and sodium fluoride solutions to prevent enamel erosion. *Journal of Dentistry* 43: 1498–1503.

22 Sundaram, G., Bartlett, D, Watson, T. (2004). Bonding to and protecting worn palatal surfaces of teeth with dentine bonding agents. *Journal of Oral Rehabiliation* 31(5): 505–509.

23 Bartlett, D., Sundaram, G., Moazzez, R. (2011). Trial of protective effect of fissure sealants, in vivo, on the palatal surfaces of anterior teeth, in patients suffering from erosion. *Journal of Dentistry* 39(1): 26–29.

24 Dahl, B.L., Krogstad, O., Karlsen, K. (1975). An alternative treatment of cases with advanced localised attrition. *Journal of Oral Rehabilitation* 2: 209–214.

25 Dahl BL, Krogstad O. (1985). Long-term observations of an increased occlusal face height obtained by a combined orthodontic/prosthetic approach. *Journal of Oral Rehabilitation* 12: 173–176.

26 Cohen, D. (2012). The truth about sports drinks. *British Medical Journal* 345: e4737.

27 Milosevic, A. (1997). Sports drinks hazard to teeth. *British Journal of Sports Medicine* 31(1): 28–30.

28 Coombes, J.S. (2005). Sports drinks and dental erosion. *American Journal of Dentistry* 18(2): 101–104.

29 Edwards, M., Creanor, S.L., Foye, R.H., Gilmour, W.H. (1999). Buffering capacities of soft drinks: the potential influence on dental erosion. *Journal of Oral Rehabilitation* 26(12): 923–927.

30 Attin, T., Weiss, K., Becker, K., Buchalla, W., Wiegand, A. (2005). Impact of modified acidic soft drinks on enamel erosion. *Oral Diseases* 11(1): 7–12.

31 Needleman, I., Ashley, P., Fine, P., et al. (2015). Oral health and elite sport performance. *British Journal of Sports Medicine* 49(1): 3–6.

7

Prevention of Sporting Dental Injuries
Peter D. Fine

7.1   Introduction

In previous chapters in this book, we have discussed the prevalence, incidence, and consequences of dental trauma, as well as how to repair fractured teeth on the short-, mid- and long-term basis. When speaking about the prevention of dental trauma it would be easy to consider the use of mouth guards and very little else. In this chapter, we look at the limited evidence to support early intervention by an orthodontist as a preventative measure, the need to educate athletes, coaches, and managers about the dental implications of a high carbohydrate diet and mouth guards. We will also mention the use of head protection as in scrumcaps (rugby), helmets (cricket), and face shields (ice hockey).

Dealing with dental trauma as a result of sporting accidents can be time-consuming for the athlete, costly, and involve a lifetime of restorative treatment, depending on the severity of the trauma. In a study by Andersson, it was reported that 13–39% of all dental traumas were related to sports [1]. The long-term prognosis for those teeth was highly dependent on prompt, accurate diagnosis being available and expedient treatment being undertaken by a well-qualified professional. The cost of this treatment is high and has been estimated to be as much as $2–5 per million inhabitants [1].

The evidence that the prevention of sporting trauma actually works is mixed. A study undertaken in Austria concluded that the appropriate design of helmets with faceguards (Figure 7.1) would reduce the incidence of facial injuries caused by cycling-related accidents [2]. Interestingly, this study compared those cycling as a mode of transport (street cyclists) with those mountain biking as a recreational pursuit. Facial bone fractures were more prevalent in mountain bikers (55% compared to 34.5%); dento-alveola trauma was more prevalent in the sample of street cyclists (58% compared to 22%); and soft tissue lesions were more common in mountain bikers (23% compared to 14%).

Mountain biking is becoming more popular, as is cycling in general. In the UK this appears to be particularly following the success of British Cycling during recent Olympic and World Championships. A study with a sample of 423 male mountain bikers from Europe revealed that 5.7% had experienced trauma to their teeth following a fall from their bike; 71.9% knew about mouth guards, but only 4% used them [3].

The introduction of mandatory mouth guards in professional rugby union in New Zealand has seen a 43% drop in the number of dental trauma cases [4]. The need for constant review of the laws, the need to identify injury trends as players become heavier, faster, and more professional, the need for

Sports Dentistry: Principles and Practice, First Edition. Edited by Peter D. Fine, Chris Louca and Albert Leung.
© 2019 John Wiley & Sons Ltd. Published 2019 by John Wiley & Sons Ltd.
Companion website: www.wiley.com/go/fine/sports_dentistry

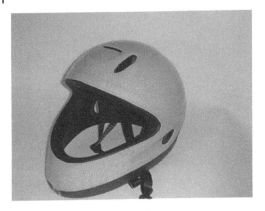

Figure 7.1 Suitable cycle helmet with faceguard.

education of players and coaches. and the need for ongoing research are all essential if we are to prevent not only trauma to the orofacial area, but all injuries. It is unrealistic to expect a complete cessation of all trauma in contact sports like rugby, hockey, basketball, and handball, but a reduction where possible is obviously beneficial to players, teams, and the future of the sport.

7.2 Concussion

In Chapter 1, we briefly discussed concussion, which is extremely topical at present. Prevention of head injuries and concussion in particular has received a great deal of media attention in the last few years and has concentrated the thoughts of journalists, coaches, athletes, players, parents, and medical colleagues [5]. There is, however, a misconception and an ill-conceived belief that the wearing of a sports mouth guard can prevent concussion. The evidence to support this idea is rather patchy and so until there is substantial evidence to support the wearing of mouth guards as a realistic, effective way of preventing concussion, as medical/dental practitioners, we should be wary of suggesting the mouth guard for this purpose. I shall consider the role of mouth guards more fully later in this chapter.

Early research suggested that concussion was sustained by 2.7% of subjects in a study comparing the use or non-use of mouth guards in sport [6]. This would suggest that the use of mouth guards was not necessary to prevent concussion; 3.1% of the sample wore a mouth guard and received concussion, whereas 2.5 % did not wear a mouth guard and received concussion. Blignaut also reported no significant difference between wearing a mouth guard or not when it came to the incidence of head and neck injuries, and more surprisingly mouth, tooth, and lip injuries [6]. This study suggested that whether you wear a mouth guard or not has no bearing on the likelihood of dental trauma. I shall consider the use of mouth guards later in this chapter.

The reporting of concussion is somewhat spasmodic. For example, McCrea et al. reported that 29.9% of respondents reported a previous history of concussion, and 15.3% reported sustaining a concussion during the current football season; of those, 47.3% reported their injury [7]. Concussions were reported most frequently to a certified athletic trainer (76.7% of reported injuries). The most common reasons for concussion not being reported included a player not thinking the injury was serious enough to warrant medical attention (66.4% of unreported injuries), not wanting to be withheld from competition (41.0%), and lack of awareness of probable concussion (36.1%). These findings reflect a higher prevalence of concussion in high school football players than previously reported in the literature. The ultimate concern associated with unreported concussion is an athlete's increased risk of cumulative or catastrophic effects from recurrent injury. Future prevention initiatives should focus on education to improve athlete awareness of the signs of concussion and potential risks of unreported injury.

While head injuries can occur in virtually any form of athletic activity, they occur most frequently in contact sports, such as football (Figure 7.2), boxing, and martial arts competitions, or from high-velocity collisions or falls in basketball, soccer, and ice hockey. The pathophysiology of concussion is less well

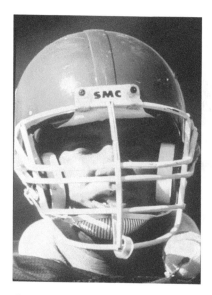

Figure 7.2 American Football helmet and mouth guard.

sports coaches, coaching education was prophetic of the ability to recognize signs and symptoms of sport-related concussion [9]. However, several misconceptions about concussion still exist, highlighting that education regarding concussion is necessary. The presence of qualified health care personnel, such as an athletic trainer, medical practitioner, or dental practitioner at the youth organization level may enhance early recognition, treatment, and referral of concussions. If in doubt, the player should be removed from the field of play and referred for further investigation.

7.3 The Role of Schools in Mouth Guard Wear

Schools have a responsibility to prevent injuries to students whilst in their care. This includes the prevention of sporting injuries whilst the students are in school or representing the school. Their duty of care extends to ensuring that students are safe during their time in school and includes facilities, sporting equipment, and activities. Many schools have made the wearing of mouth guards compulsory during contact sports in particular, and have invited individuals or manufacturers into school to provide suitable mouth guards.

In Australia there is a tradition of early involvement of children in contact sports. However, there is little research to illustrate the compulsory value of mouth guards in schools. Previous studies of high school Rugby Union players in New Zealand have shown that between 13 and 15% had previously sustained dental injury, while between 30 and 37% wore mouth guards regularly. One hundred and thirty Rugby Union football players attending a large high school in Brisbane participated in this survey [10]. All believed in the safety value of mouth guards in rugby. As a result of all of the players in the four open teams

understood than that of severe head injury, and it has received less attention as a result. Kelly et al. described a high school football player who died of diffuse brain swelling after repeated concussions without loss of consciousness [8]. Guidelines have been developed to reduce the risk of such serious catastrophic outcomes after concussion in sports. Whilst these fatalities are rare, we need to be aware of their possibility and advise the sportsman/woman of potential risks.

Clear guidelines are also presented as to when to discontinue collision sport competition for a protracted period of time, i.e. the remainder of the season, after multiple concussions. Because of the concern for the second impact syndrome, the requirement to never allow an athlete with post-concussion syndrome symptoms to return to competition needs to be emphasised to athletes and coaches. We need additional research on the cumulative effects of concussion to prevent the long-term effects of repeated blows to the head.

There appears to be a need for more education of coaches regarding concussion. Mcleod et al., revealed that, among youth and the bulk of players in the four under-age teams wearing mouth guards, the incidence of dental injury was very low, approximately 4%.

There is a growing realisation that by encouraging 'Health Promoting Schools', which generate an atmosphere of developing a range of complementary policies and actions to promote the health and wellbeing of students, teachers, and the wider community, by focusing on the effect of the social and physical environment on health, particularly dental trauma problems can be prevented [11]. In relation to the prevention of dental trauma, including and beyond the sporting context, a wide range of actions and policies are possible: (i) personal and social education aimed at developing life skills, for example conflict resolution, dealing with relationship issues, and health skills in relation to misuse of drugs and alcohol; (ii) developing a robust school policy on bullying and violence between students, creating a positive atmosphere for social support; (iii) monitoring play areas, sports fields, sports equipment, and security; (iv) schools need to extend their health policy to educating staff in first aid measures; (v) there should be a schools policy on wearing of mouth guards, which are accessible to all students; (vi) schools should have a well-documented policy for dealing with dental trauma; correct procedures in place for emergency treatment, screening programmes, staff training, and support from healthcare professionals on prevention of dental trauma, this last aspect being part of the remit of a sports dentist.

7.4   The Use of Helmets in Preventing Sporting Trauma

Alpine skiing and snowboarding are increasingly popular winter sports and are enjoyed by several hundred million people worldwide. However, the wearing of a helmet is not compulsory, but is associated with reduced

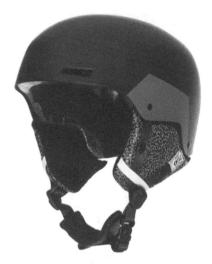

Figure 7.3 Ski helmet.

risk of head injury among snowboarders and alpine skiers (Figure 7.3). Head injury is the most frequent reason for hospital admission and the most common cause of death among skiers and snowboarders, with an 8% fatality rate among those admitted to hospital with head injuries [12]. In cycling, case-control studies indicate that helmets reduce the risk of head injury, and helmets are strongly advocated to prevent head injuries in cycling and in-line skating. Helmets are also mandatory for competitive skiers in the Fédération Internationale de Ski (FIS) World Cup events in all disciplines [13]. The use of helmet is generally low among recreational skiers and snowboarders, (although increasing), although their use is higher among children. Opponents of mandatory helmet use even claim that helmets may increase the risk because they may lead to a reduced field of vision, impaired hearing, or increased speed through a false feeling of security, and thus increase the incidence of collisions, the cause of many severe injuries [14]. Another argument against helmet use is the uncertainty about whether it might cause a higher risk of cervical spine injuries, through a guillotine effect of the heavy helmet, especially in children [15,16].

7.5 Early Intervention Orthodontics

There is little scientific evidence to support the idea that early intervention orthodontics to reduce a severe overjet is beneficial in preventing sporting trauma [17]. However, it would seem logical that by reducing a 9 mm overjet and giving the vulnerable upper central incisors some protection from the lips would be beneficial (See Figure 7.4).

In a study of 1367 children undertaken in an orthodontic practice, it was reported that 10.3% of these patients had suffered from dental trauma before the onset of orthodontic treatment. The highest prevalence of dental trauma was in the 11–15 years age group, corresponding to the dental developmental stage of the late mixed dentition. The most frequently affected teeth were the maxillary

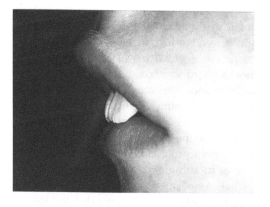

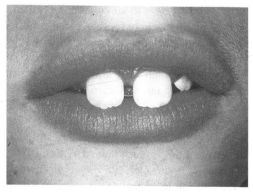

Figure 7.4 **Severe overjet and incompetent lip morphology.**

central incisors (79.6%), and the most common types of trauma were fracture of enamel–dentine without pulpal involvement (42.7%) and fracture of enamel (33.8%). Compared to patients with normal overjet and adequate lip coverage, the frequency of dental trauma was significantly higher in patients with increased overjet and adequate lip coverage (P = 0.028) or with increased overjet and inadequate lip coverage (P = 0.003). The results of this study indicate that a significant percentage of candidates for orthodontic treatment, and especially those with increased overjet and inadequate lip coverage, suffer trauma to their permanent incisors before the onset of orthodontic treatment. It might also be concluded that preventive orthodontic treatment of such patients should be initiated and completed before the age of 11, i.e. in the early to middle mixed dentition stage [18].

The evidence suggests that providing early orthodontic treatment to deal with prominent front teeth is more effective in reducing the incidence of incisal trauma than providing a course of orthodontic treatment when the child is in early adolescence. There does not appear to be any other advantage to providing early treatment when compared to treatment in adolescence [19].

In a study looking at the prevalence of trauma to the permanent dentition of the child population, it was shown that children with an overjet of 6 mm or more had a four times higher risk of trauma than did those with a 'normal' overjet [20]. They concluded that early intervention of orthodontic treatment could lead to a reduction in the amount of dental trauma. This study also highlighted the upper central incisors as those teeth most likely to be traumatised.

So, although the evidence is not overwhelming, it would seem sensible to at least consider early orthodontic interventions, even if it means the child would have to undergo a further course of treatment later on during adolescence. I shall consider the role of the mouth guard in preventing dental trauma later in the chapter, but the implications of trauma to vulnerable teeth prior to ortho- dontic intervention should be considered. The main arguments against using mouth guards during orthodontic treatment seem to be based on the continually changing shape of the dental arch and the cost implica- tions of making new mouth guards on a reg- ular basis, i.e. every two to three months. Both these challenges can be overcome by suggesting that the parent purchases a good- quality heat-cured mouth guard in a sports store or on-line, and brings it into the dentist, who can mould it to the individual before relining the trough of the mouth guard with a soft lining material. This can easily be replaced when the mouth guard becomes ill- fitting. Care needs to be taken in using this technique to block out undercuts and ortho- dontic brackets/arch wires with a soft wax prior to relining. By using a heat-cured appli- ance that has a good shape to start with, a close-fitting, comfortable mouth guard can be adapted to the ever-changing shape of the dental arch, thus avoiding the need to purchase a new custom-made mouth guard every few months, and allowing the young athlete to pursue their sport of choice. At the conclusion of orthodontic treatment, final study casts should be given to the patient as a record of their final tooth relationship, occlusion, and appearance.

7.6 Mouth Guards

The role of a mouth guard is clearly to protect the teeth, but there are claims that mouth guards protect the temporomandibular joint (TMJ) and prevent neurological trauma (concussion). There is evidence that a well- constructed mouth guard will protect the temporomandibular joint from trauma, but the evidence on whether mouth guards can be relied upon to prevent concussion is very sketchy. The sports shops are full of a myriad of designs of mouth guard, each claiming to be the latest and best option. The history of mouth guards is somewhat unclear; references have gone back to the turn of the twentieth century, when it would appear that boxing was the first sport in which mouth guards were used. It has been reported that in 1890, Woolfe Krause, a London dentist, developed a mouth guard or 'gum shield' to protect boxers from debilitating lip lacerations. These early gum shields were made from gutta percha and were held in place by the individual clenching their teeth together. The next development saw the use of vella rubber to construct the gum shield. Dentists then developed the mouth guard over a period of years until, in 1927, a boxing match between Mike McTigue and Jack Sharkey in the USA, which was clearly being won by McTigue, was stopped following the chipping of a front tooth, which resulted in a laceration of the lip. Mouth guards then became com- monplace for boxers. Three years after this famous fight, Dr Clearance Mayer, a dentist and a boxing inspector published an article on mouth guards, explaining how custom-made mouth guards could be fashioned from impres- sions using wax and rubber.

In 1947 the first clear acrylic resin mouth guard was made, which fitted over the upper and lower teeth, but was considered to be much more unobtrusive. The value of this mouth guard was recognised by other sports and very soon afterwards Dick Perry, a basket- ball player, became the first athlete to use an acrylic mouth guard. Frankie Albert, the quar- terback for the San Francisco 49ers, was the first known professional athlete to wear this type of mouth guard. By 1960 the American Dental Association (ADA) had researched mouth guards and recommended the use of latex mouth guards in all contact sports and by 1962 all high school football players in the US were required to wear a mouth guard.

In the mid 1990s technology was developed for fabricating high heat and pressure lami- nated mouth guards. Different thicknesses were produced to allow for the ideal thickness and allowing for reduction in thickness. The evolution of materials used to fabricate cus- tom-made mouth guards has led to the current polyvinyl acetate–polyethylene co-polymer (PVA–PE) laminate, which can be laminated to itself using vacuum pressure (see Figure 7.5).

It is assumed that simply wearing a mouth guard of any form of construction will

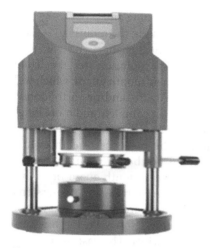

Figure 7.5 The Drufomat machine for fabricating custom-made mouth guards.

prevent trauma to the teeth. There is, however, mixed evidence in the literature to support this assumption. De Wet reported that there were no injuries to the teeth when a custom-made mouth guard was worn in junior athletes, but that there were 21.3% tooth injuries when a mouth guard was not worn [21]. In addition, De Wet described damage to lips (18.7%) and other soft tissues (6.7%) with a mouth guard, whereas 41.3% and 16%, respectively, were traumatised without a mouth guard being worn.

Further evidence as to the effectiveness of wearing a mouth guard was reported when looking at dental trauma during the Canadian Games; it was observed that 'none of the athletes who sustained injuries was wearing a mouth guard' [22]. Jolly et al. observed that when a mouth guard was not worn during football games, the likelihood of a fractured or avulsed tooth was at least twice that when a mouth guard was worn [23].

From this data it would appear that the wearing of a mouth guard prevented trauma to teeth and reduced the amount of trauma to the soft tissues. This study only looked at junior athletes and only mentioned the use of custom-made mouth guards; we do not know if the same is true in other age groups and with other types of mouth guard.

By contrast, a study looking at mouth guard wear relative to mouth, tooth, and lip injuries, showed that 95.4% of mouth guard wearers did not get injuries and that 95.3% of non-wearers also did not get injuries [6]. This would suggest that there was very little difference between wearers and non-wearers in terms of the amount of trauma to dental, oral, and labial tissues. In a study looking at the injury rate of wearers and non-wearers with respect to brain, oral, and dental injuries, a slight difference in dental injuries was shown, but no significant difference was seen when looking at brain and oral injuries, whether a mouth guard was worn or not [24]. This finding once again brings into question the value of wearing a mouth guard for sports.

In recent years it has fallen upon schools to make the wearing of mouth guards for contact sports compulsory. The influence that professional athletes have on children desperate to follow in their heroes' footsteps should not be under-rated. Elite athletes can have both a positive and negative effect on children and the wearing of mouth guards is a prime example. In order to set a 'good' example, the elite athletes need to be knowledgeable about why they wear a mouth guard, rather than just wearing it. In a study looking at the knowledge professional rugby players have with regard to the benefits of wearing a mouth guard, and comparing with that of children and parents starting out in sport, the professionals have a much greater understanding of the benefits of wearing a mouth guard. Parents agreed that children should wear a mouth guard for contact sport as soon as possible, but few actually did [25].

Sports shops and on-line suppliers offer a wide range of mouth guards, which fall into one of three categories: stock mouth guards, boil and bite mouth guards, and custom-made mouth guards. The stock mouth guards just fit the mouth of the wearer where they touch. They are made from either rubber or polyvinyl and come in small, medium, or large. However, very little can be done to adjust their fit, they are bulky, make breathing and talking difficult, and would appear to provide a limited amount of protection. Boil and bite mouth guards are, as their name suggests, made from a thermoplastic material, which is placed into hot water to soften and then adapted in the mouth by the athlete biting into the plastic to fit the occlusal surface, modifying with the tongue, and sucking it into place. These mouth guards do fit a little more comfortably than stock mouth guards, but are limited by their shape and the amount of hard tissue they cover. The advantage of this type of mouth guard is its relatively cheap cost and that adaptability to a changing dentition is possible by resoftening and remoulding the mouth guard. Historically, this type of mouth guard was used by 47.7% of boxers in 1982, before the advent of custom-made mouth guards.

The custom-made mouth guard is thought to be the most effective in terms of protecting teeth and the tempero-mandibular joints. These appliances are individually designed and manufactured, either in the dental practice or a commercial dental laboratory. Accurate upper and lower impressions of the teeth are taken in a suitable impression material (e.g. alginate) using an appropriate impression tray (rigid metal). The custom-made mouth guard fits comfortably around the upper anterior teeth, covers the pre-maxilla, extends posteriorly to include the first permanent molar teeth and extends 10 mm from the palatal gingival margin into the palate to aid retention and help dissipate any shock.

The reluctance to wearing a mouth guard could be due to several factors. There is a perception that mouth guards are uncomfortable, the player cannot speak or breathe properly with it in place, and that the child loses it too easily. A significant barrier to the use of mouth guards is the perceived cost. With the dentition of the child constantly changing, the awareness is that a mouth guard will need to be replaced every few months.

In order to overcome this problem, a stock mouth guard bought from a sports shop can be regularly relined in the dental chair by the practitioner, using a soft denture relining material. When the dentition changes in either its relative position or in the number of teeth present, the practitioner can simply

remove the soft relining and replace it with a new layer, thus making the mouth guard serviceable until the next change. This is an economic and quick solution to the child growing out of their mouth guard, which will suffice until growth and/or orthodontic treatment has been complete and more long-lasting device can be made. Orthodontic treatment and the presence of orthodontic brackets should not be a reason for a child either to not have a mouth guard or not to play their favourite sport. Before impressions for the mouth guard are taken, it is essential to 'block-out' with a soft wax, the brackets and orthodontic wires. The vast majority of trauma to teeth occurs to the upper incisors [26], so the early reduction of an increased overjet should be considered. This should be done in consultation with an orthodontic specialist and following radiographic examination, particularly to ascertain where the developing upper canines are situated in order to prevent further crowding of these teeth. Where a young athlete has a lower fixed appliance in place or indeed if there is thought to be the need for protection to lower restorations from trauma, a lower, or upper and lower mouth guard might be considered. Figure 7.6 illustrates a basic stock mouth guard designed to cover both the upper and lower dentition, but with very little retention, comfort, or protection.

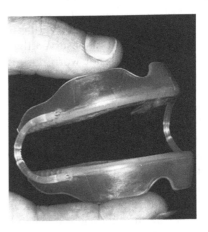

Figure 7.6 Stock mouth guard for upper and lower teeth.

7.6.1 Impressions for a Mouth Guard

In order to give the dental technician sufficient information to make a suitable mouth guard, upper and lower alginate impressions are needed. The impressions should include the teeth as far back as the first molar, the pre-maxilla, labial sulcus, palatal tissues, and occlusal surfaces of the teeth. The impressions should be as accurate as possible and if recorded in a hydrophilic material like dental alginate, should be cast, in hard stone, within the hour, to prevent distortion. Alginate is an irreversible hydrocolloid impression material that is ideal for these impressions, but needs to be treated with care. Metal trays should be used to give adequate support to the material, if sending to a laboratory minimal disinfection requirements should be adhered to, and the casts should be set on a hinge articulator. Provided that the inter-cuspal position is obvious, no bite registration is needed. It is essential to liaise with the dental technician and inform him/her about the shape you want the mouth guard, how many layers of laminate you want fused together, which sport the patient is playing, and any areas, such as erupting teeth, that need to be accounted for. The custom-made mouth guard should be 5 mm thickness anteriorly and 3–4 mm thickness posteriorly. Each layer of laminate is normally 3 mm thick (although thicker layers can be used), so for most sports two layers is sufficient; optimal thicknesses can be achieved by allowing for some shrinkage during the processing of the mouth guard. The mouth guard should cover the teeth as far back as the first molar, cover the labial, palatal, and incisal/occlusal surfaces and palatally extend to 10 mm beyond the gingival margin. Labially, the mouth guard should protect the pre-maxilla by extending into that area (see Figures 7.7 and 7.8).

This design has been shown to be comfortable, functional and most important wearable. As can be seen in Figure 7.9, the lower teeth engage in the occlusal surface of the mouth guard, which gives the lower incisors some degree of protection, but also prevents trauma to the mandible and temporomandibular joint following a blow to the side of the mandible, by supporting the lower jaw. By setting the casts on a simple hinge articulator it is possible to achieve this extra protection whilst maintaining the correct thickness of material. Obviously the colour of the mouth guard is an individual preference that can be accommodated with this system.

When constructing mouth guards for patients playing certain sports like hockey, lacrosse, and ice hockey, the potential danger from a hard stick or ball/puck, means that you may need to consider using more than two layers of laminate to increase the thickness and therefore the degree of protection. By using a system that employs a machine like the Drufomat, as many layers can be

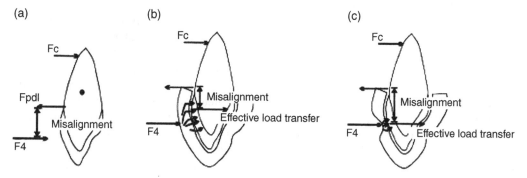

Figure 7.7 (a) Forces (F) acting on a tooth with and without the use of mouthguard during a soft object collision. (b) Forces (F) acting on a tooth with a high stiffness mouthguard. (c) Forces (F) acting on a tooth with a low stiffness mouthguard.

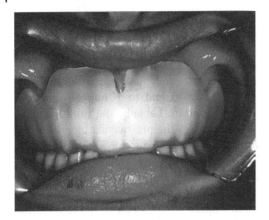

Figure 7.8 Ideal shape for mouth guard, labial view.

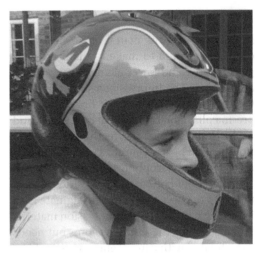

Figure 7.10 Cycle helmet.

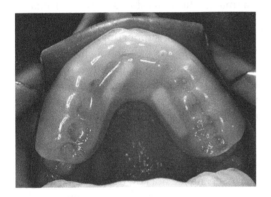

Figure 7.9 Ideal shape for mouth guard, occlusal view.

bonded together as you wish; but a word of caution – the thicker the mouth guard, the more stretched the upper lip becomes and the more likely that is of splitting, particularly from a punch (boxing), elbow (basketball), or simple collision (hockey).

7.7 Helmets

To prevent or minimise head or brain injuries in sport, for athletes such as boxers, cricketers, footballers, cyclists, skiers, baseball players, and participants in motorsports, helmets are mandatory or recommended (Figure 7.10). These helmets are specifically designed and rigorously tested according to the impacts of different types of sports.

A helmet designed for cricket may not be suitable for a cyclist or boxer. The player's helmet should fit well in order to prevent damage from wearing it.

The use of protective helmets in sport can prevent serious injuries to the head, jaws, and face.

7.8 Face Shields

The introduction of face shields, particularly in ice hockey, led to a reduction in the number of facial injuries. Benson et al. compared the effectiveness of full face shield and half face shields in ice hockey players, which it was speculated may increase their risk of concussions and neck injuries, thus offsetting the benefits of protection from dental, facial, and ocular injuries [27]. Of 319 athletes who wore full face shields, 195 (61.6%) had at least one injury during the study season, whereas of 323 who wore half face shields, 204 (63.2%) were injured. The risk of sustaining a facial laceration and dental injury was 2.31 (95% confidence interval [CI], 1.53–3.48; $P < 0.001$) and 9.90 (95% CI, 1.88–52.1; $P = 0.007$) times greater, respectively, for players wearing half vs. full face shields. No statistically significant risk differences were found for neck injuries, concussion, or other injuries, although time lost from participation because of concussion was significantly greater in the half shield group (P < 0.001), than in the group wearing full shields.

These data provide evidence that the use of full face shields is associated with significantly reduced risk of sustaining facial and dental injuries without an increase in the risk of neck injuries, concussions, or other injuries.

Figure 7.11 illustrates a half face shield in toughened Perspex, for visibility, and a metallic grill for protection of the nasal and oral areas. Prior to the introduction of this protection the loss of upper front teeth was

considered a consequence of playing professional hockey and indeed some considered the loss of front teeth to be a 'badge of honour'.

The grills worn by cricketers around the world have evolved to protect the facial area and are continually being modified to cover additional vulnerable areas, e.g. the mastoid bones. Figure 7.12 illustrates that despite continuing efforts to increase the level of protection, the grill on this cricket helmet leaves the eyes vulnerable to trauma. The batsman/batswoman needs to be able to see the ball clearly and therefore a space is left in the grill, which leaves the eyes exposed.

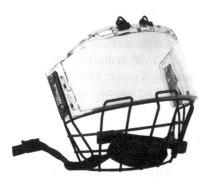

Figure 7.11 Ice hockey half face shield and grill.

7.9 Education About Diet

In Chapter 8 we deal with the specificity of nutrition with respect to athletes generally, but with elite athletes particularly in mind. Most of our patients need to be reminded about the potential detrimental effects of sugars in our diets, particularly from the point of view of dental caries, as well as the need for good oral practices. Arguably, elite athletes are in greater need of education due to their continuous consumption of sugary

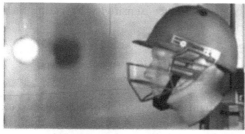
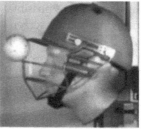
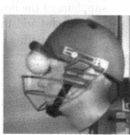
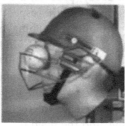

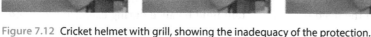

Figure 7.12 Cricket helmet with grill, showing the inadequacy of the protection.

snacks, sports drinks, and energy bars/gels, all of which are considered necessary to fulfil their need for a large calorific intake. It is estimated that an Olympic oarsman needs to consume 7000–8000 calories per day to maintain their level of fitness prior to a rowing regatta. Without tackling the larger and more pervasive socio-economic changes that appear to be preconditions for change, there are serious challenges in modifying some behaviours to effect changes in lifestyle [27]. The individual nature of oral health education means that education is time-consuming, expensive, and constantly needs reinforcing. It may be possible to include oral health promotion within the remit of an integrated approach to health education, thus reducing the small number of risk factors, which may have a significant impact on a large number of diseases at a low cost, and greater efficiency and effectiveness than a disease-specific approach.

A knowledge of nutritional goals is the first stage in developing appropriate eating strategies, and a change in attitude to eating may also be necessary. Changing dietary habits is therefore a slow, difficult process and in many cases athletes will require professional help and support to steer them in the correct direction [28].

It is also worth reinforcing the message about diet on as many occasions as possible. These can include during pre-season screening (See Chapter 10), on a one-to-one level in the dental surgery, by holding sessions designed to educate athletes, and by teaching our medical colleagues what is good oral health and the potential pitfalls of poor oral health. We need to consider the role of sugars in the caries (dental decay) process, the role of acidity in foods/drinks with respect to dental erosion, the role of clenching and grinding teeth that have already suffered from some erosive tooth surface loss, and the role of preventative regimes such as the use of fluoride as a toothpaste or gel, the importance of good oral hygiene to regularly remove dental plaque, and the need for routine dental check-ups.

Athletes who compete in endurance sports, triathlon, marathon running, cycling, and Nordic skiing need to consume large quantities of carbohydrates to support their training and competition, to help repair damaged tissues, and to replace sugar levels to fuel muscles. These athletes are likely to continuously eat carbohydrates during a day of training or competition, thus exposing their dentition to constant bombardment from sugars. These athletes need to be advised as to what preventative measures they should take: brushing of teeth and gingival tissues, but not immediately following a sugar attack, the importance of hydration, and the use of fluoride as a toothpaste, gel, or in the form of Recaldent™. Recaldent is derived from the milk protein, casein. For many years it has been known that milk and its derivatives have a tooth-protective effect. Research has shown that this activity is due to a part of the casein protein called casein phosphopeptide (or CPP), which carries calcium and phosphate ions in the form of amorphous calcium phosphate (or ACP).

Recaldent has an active ingredient of 10% CPP-ACP. It acts as a saliva replacement/substitute and helps to re-establish the oral balance following an acid attack. There is evidence that it will aid in re-establishing an artificial pellicle to protect tooth enamel and helps to reduce sensitivity by acting as a desensitizer.

7.10 Sports Drinks

The main functions of sports drinks are to: (1) supply a source of carbohydrate that can supplement the limited stores of glycogen in the muscles and the liver; (2) replace losses through sweating; and (3) reduce the problems associated with dehydration during training and competition. This is obviously more significant in hot climates, but needs to be taken seriously at all times and at all levels of sport. The ability of a sports drink to maintain fluid balance during exercise is dependent upon the rates of fluid ingestion, gastric emptying, and intestinal absorption. Glycogen-compromised individuals, for example athletes taking part in extreme sports like ultra-marathons and triathlons, undoubtedly benefit from consumption of carbohydrate-containing sports drinks. However, improvement of performance in those athletes with sufficient levels of glycogen is less certain, for example soccer players. Consumption of a sports drink during intermittent exercise, as well as prior to and during prolonged exercise, appears to improve performance. The role of sports drinks has been widened to include the replacement of essential minerals, carbohydrates, and salts. A study undertaken by Coombes and Hamilton, reviewed articles to evaluate the effectiveness of commercially available sports drinks. They asked two questions: (1) will consuming a sports drink be beneficial to performance? and (2i) do different sports drinks vary in their effectiveness? [29] They considered the composition of commercially available sports drinks, examined the rationale for using them, and critically reviewed the vast number of studies that have investigated the effectiveness of sports drinks on performance. They focused on the drinks that contain low carbohydrate concentrations (<10%) and are marketed for general consumption before and during exercise rather than those with carbohydrate concentrations >10%, which are intended for carbohydrate loading. Coombes and Hamilton [29] concluded that: (1) because of variations in drink composition and research design, much of the sports drinks research from the past cannot be applied directly to the effectiveness of currently available sports drinks; (2) in studies where a practical protocol has been used along with a currently available sports beverage, there is evidence to suggest that consuming a sports drinks will improve performance compared with consuming a placebo beverage; and (3) there is little evidence that any one sports drink is superior to any of the others.

From the findings of this study we can conclude that the marketing of commercially available sports drinks is very important to the manufacturers, as there is little difference in their individual effectiveness. The marketing of sports drinks is geared to persuading the purchaser (or the parent) that the individual manufacturer's sports drink will help the athlete to run faster, throw further, and lift heavier weights, and is often supported by elite athletes who endorse the product with their name and/or tales of success. This may sound like a somewhat sceptical comment, but it is borne out by studies that have been undertaken looking at milk as a suitable recovery drink following exertion/exercise, particularly following resistance training and endurance sports.

There is currently only limited research, but milk appears to be an effective post-resistance exercise beverage that results in favourable acute alterations in protein metabolism. Milk consumption acutely increases muscle protein synthesis, leading to an improved net muscle protein balance. Furthermore, when post-exercise milk consumption is combined with resistance training (12 weeks minimum), greater increases in muscle hypertrophy and lean mass have been observed. Although research with milk is limited, there is some evidence to suggest that milk may be an effective post-exercise drink for endurance activities. Low-fat milk has been shown to be as effective, if not more so, than commercially available sports drinks as a rehydration drink. Milk represents a more nutrient dense drink for individuals who partake in strength and endurance activities, compared to traditional sports drinks. Bovine low-fat liquid milk is a safe and effective post-exercise beverage for most individuals, except for those who are lactose intolerant [30].

There is some evidence to suggest that milk contains 'quantities of IGF-1 and other growth factors which are prohibited and can influence the outcome of anti-doping tests. Therefore, WADA does not recommend the ingestion of this product' [31]. The World Anti-Doping Agency (WADA) is responsible for the drug testing of all athletes worldwide, whether in or out of competition. The agency was established in 1999 as an international independent agency composed and funded equally by the sport movement and governments of the world. Its key activities include scientific research, education, development of anti-doping capabilities, and monitoring of the World Anti Doping Code – the document harmonizing anti-doping policies in all sports and all countries.

It will be interesting to see whether milk becomes a substance added to the banned list along with other 'drugs' such as anabolic agents, beta-2-agonists, and hormone and metabolic regulators. As dentists we need to be aware of the substances on WADA's list in case we should inadvertently prescribe such a substance for patients who may be being regularly tested. However, it should be noted that the ultimate responsibility rests with the athlete, who, if they are in any doubt about a medicament that they may need for health reasons, can apply for a 'Therapeutic Use Exemption'.

7.11   Prevention of Dental Diseases

In Chapter 10 we look at the role of regular dental screening and its value for elite athletes. It has long been established that regular dental examinations are a good way of spotting disease and either dealing with or monitoring it. This is especially true for elite athletes, who often have a diet rich in carbohydrates, consume large quantities of sports drinks, have little time to visit the dentist as they are travelling, and who may have sacrificed early age dental care for a training session or competition. Very often we only get to see these athletes when they have a problem, when they are off to a training session or competition, or when the club medical team call us in. It is important, whenever we can, to spread the word about preventative dentistry in the form of good oral hygiene, being aware of good dietary practices, education about periodontal (gum) issues, and the use of fluoride mouthwashes and

toothpaste. It is unlikely that a busy athlete is going to change their oral hygiene behaviour just because the dentist mentions it is good for oral health and looking after their teeth and gums for the future.

Elite athletes do not respond to health measures that are not going to have an immediate and significant impact on their performance. So if you can tell an Olympic sprinter that if he/she improves their oral care they will improve their time for the 100 metres, and have evidence to prove it, then fine. At present, despite lots of anecdotal evidence, we don't have scientific proof of the fact. What we can do, without breaking confidentiality, is to report the experiences of other athletes, in particular how a dental issue interrupted training or performance and that we should all learn from that. Trauma in a contact sport is something that a few athletes feel will not happen to them, but by showing them the consequences of a traumatic incident to another athlete we may be able to change their mind to look at prevention more seriously.

7.12   Performance-enhancing Mouth Guards

This chapter has been concerned with the prevention of tooth tissue loss, either acutely as a result of trauma, chronically through erosion and abrasion. It would not be complete, however, without mentioning the use of 'performance-enhancing mouth guards' (Figure 7.13). The use of these custom-made mouthpieces is becoming more prevalent, particularly in weight strengthening exercises, for golfers, and during training sessions. I have included a small section here on the use of performance-enhancing mouth guards as an effective way of improving/enhancing sporting performance. Some authors claim that mouth guards can enhance athletic performance [32,33], although this view is not universally accepted. The principle behind these mouth guards, which are custom made, often fitted on the lower jaw,

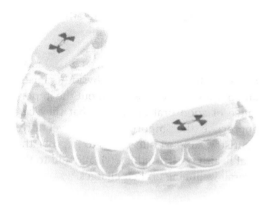

Figure 7.13 Performance-enhancing mouth guard.

and still in the development phase, is to reduce the levels of cortisol, the stress hormone produced in the facial muscles as the athlete clenches their teeth together. According to Duddy et al., 'Teeth clench in response to elevated stress levels. This clenching mechanism completes a circuit and signals the brain to begin a complex series of responses in the hypothalamic–pituitary–adrenal (HPA) axis. As a result, the adrenal glands release adrenaline, noradrenaline, and cortisol, all enabling the body's stress response. Adrenaline increases blood pressure, reaction time, and heart rate and sends blood to the muscles. Cortisol releases glucose, to supply the brain and muscles with immediate energy. However, at excessively high levels and particularly for long periods, the endocrine system is affected negatively. High cortisol levels limit peripheral vision, decrease metabolism, cause fatigue, reduce muscle-building, and suppress the immune system. Therefore, when stress becomes excessive, both performance and health are adversely affected. A properly designed oral appliance which prevents the teeth from occluding prevents the completion of the clenching mechanism' [34].

The evidence to support both this view and the use of performance-enhancing mouth guards both during competition and in training is far from conclusive. Further randomised controlled trials need to be undertaken to see if the principle is sound in practice, and if so whether a mouth guard designed for protection against trauma would fulfil the same role as a speciality mouth guard for performance enhancement.

There is also some evidence that a carefully constructed performance-enhancing mouth guard can ease problems of muscular/skeletal imbalance in athletes. This is particularly seen in some junior golfers, who develop an imbalance through their shoulders, back, hips, and lower limbs, resulting in reduced performance. It is thought that by wearing such an appliance, the jaw can be in harmony with the neck muscles and in turn result in the shoulders, back, hips, and lower limbs being bilaterally equal, therefore preventing a dominant side of the skeleton reducing harmony. As yet there is little scientific evident to substantiate this idea, but this is the direction that preventative dentistry is moving in the future. If by preventing an imbalance occurring or by redressing an existing imbalance in the facial musculature, we can prevent more serious skeletal issues in all athletes, then this is surely a major impact that sports dentistry can have on future safety and wellbeing of both elite and serious amateur athletes.

7.13 Conclusion

The role of dentistry in preventing damage to the dentition of our athletes can play several roles. Mouth guards, and properly constructed, wearable mouth guards are a significant move in the right direction. Whilst the wearing of a mouth guard is by no means a universal occurrence in all contact sports and the evidence for the use of mouth guards is not overwhelming, on balance the use of such a preventative appliance should be recommended rather than legislated for. All dentists are encouraged to adopt a preventative approach to their clinical work and sports dentists are no exception. When it comes to athletes our concerns about prevention move beyond those that we have for our other patients, due to the intensity of their training, their diets, their irregular attendance for advice, and the greater potential for trauma, particularly in contact sports. Education of the individual athletes about the importance of good oral health is an ongoing process. Continually re-emphasising the need for good oral hygiene, regular dental inspections, and seeking advice sooner rather than later with a minor dental issue (before it becomes a major problem), will contribute to preventing oral health problems and could mean the elite athlete winning a medal at the next Olympic Games, or failing to do so by the smallest of margins (see Chapter 9). We also need to educate coaches, trainers, sports physiotherapists, and our medical colleagues about the importance of good oral health, so that they can appreciate the importance of preventative dentistry, support our efforts to improve the oral health of their athlete(s), and add to the overall wellbeing of their charges.

References

1 Andersson, L. (2013). Epidemiology of traumatic dental injuries. *Paediatric Dentistry* 35(2): 102–105.

2 Gassner, R.J., Hackl, W., Tuli, T., Fink, L., Waldhart, E. (1999). Differential profile of facial injuries among mountainbikers compared with bicyclists. *Journal of Traumatology.* 47(1): 50–54.

3 Muller, K.E., Persic, R., Pohl, Y., Krastl, G., Fillipi, A. (2008). Dental injuries in mountain biking: a survey in Switzerland, Austria, Germany and Italy. *Dental Traumatology.* 24(5): 522–527.

4 Murray, A., Murray, I.R., Robson, J. (2014). Faster, higher, stronger: keeping an evolving sport safe. *British Journal of Sports Medicine* 48(2):73–74.

5 Patricios, J.S., Makdissi, M. (2014). The sports concussion picture: fewer 'pixels', more HD. *British Journal of Sports Medicine.* 48(2): 71–72.

6 Blignaut, J.B., Carstens, I.L., Lombard, C.J. (1987). Injuries sustained in rugby by wearers and non-wearers of mouthguards. *British Journal of Sports Medicine* 21(2): 5–7.

7 McCrea, M., Hammeke, T., Olsen, G., Leo, P., Guskiewicz, K.T.C. (2004). Unreported concussion in high school football players: implications for prevention. *Clinical Journal of Sport Medicine* 14(1): 13–17.

8 Kelly, J.P., Nichols, J.S., Filley, C.M., et al. (1991). Concussion in sports: guidelines for the prevention of catastrophic outcome. *Journal of the American Medical Association* 266(20): 2867–2869.

9 McLeod, V., Schwartz, T.C., Bay, C.M.S., Curtis, R. (2007). Sport-related concussion misunderstandings among youth coaches. *Clinical Journal of Sport Medicine* 17(2): 140–142.

10 Chapman, P.J., Nasserr, B.P. (1996). Prevalence of orofacial injuries and use of mouthguards in high school Rugby Union. *Australian Dental Journal* 41(4): 252–255.

11 World Health Organisation. (1998). *Health Promotion Schools: A Healthy Setting for Living, and Learning*WHO, Geneva.

12 Sulheim, S., Holme, I., Ekeland, A. et al. (2006). Helmet use and risk of head injuries in alpine skiers and snowboarders. *Journal of the American Medical Association* 295(8): 919–924.

13 Torjussen, J., Bahr, R. (2006). Injuries among elite snowboarders (FIS Snowboard World Cup). *British Journal of Sports Medicine* 40: 230–234.

14 Levy, A.S., Smith, R.H. (2000). Neurologic injuries in skiers and snowboarders. *Seminars in Neurology* 20: 233–245.

15 Hagel, B.E., Pless, I.B., Goulet, C., Platt, R.W., Robitaille, Y. (2005). Effectiveness of helmets in skiers and snowboarders: case-control and case crossover study. *British Medical Journal* 330: 281.

16 Deibert, M.C., Aronsson, D.D., Johnson, R.J., Ettlinger, C.F., Shealy, J.E. (1998).

Skiing injuries in children, adolescents, and adults. *Journal of Bone Joint Surgery American Volume* 80: 25–32.

17 Welbury, R. (2003). Prevention of dental trauma. In: *The Prevention of Oral Disease* (ed. Murray, J.J., Nunn, J.H., Steele, J.G.). Oxford University Press, Oxford, UK.

18 Bauss, O., Rohling, J., Schwestka-Polly, R. (2004). Prevelence of traumatic injuries to the permanent incisors in candidates for orthodontic treatment. *Dental Traumatology* 20(2): 61–66.

19 Thiruvenkatachari, B., Harrison, J.E., Worthington, H.V., O'Brien, K.D. (2013). Orthodontic treatment for prominent upper front teeth (Class II malocclusion) in children. *Cochrane Database of Systematic Reviews* 11: CD003452.

20 Schatz, J.P., Hakberg, M., Ostini, E., Kiliaridis, S. (2013). Prevalence of traumatic injuries to permanent dentition and its association with overjet in a Swiss child population. *Dental Traumatology* 29(2): 110–114.

21 De Wet, F.A. (1981). The prevention of orofacial sports injuries in the adolescent. *International Dental Journal* 31(4): 313–319.

22 Lee-Knight, C.T., Harrison, E.L., Price, C.J. (1992). Dental injuries at the 1989 Canadian Games: an epidemiological study. *Journal of Canadian Dental Association* 58: 810–815.

23 Jolly, K.A., Messer, L.B., Manton, D. (1996). Promotion of mouth guards among amateur football players in Victoria. *Australian New Zealand Journal of Public Health* 20: 630–639.

24 Labella, C.R., Smith, B.W., Sigurdsson, A. (2002). Effect of mouthguards on dental injuries and concussions in college basketball. *Medical Science and Sports Exercise* 34(1): 41–44.

25 Chatterjee, M., Hilton, I. (2007). A comparison of the attitudes and beliefs of professional rugby players from one club and parents of children playing rugby at an adjacent amateur club to the wearing of mouth guards. *Primary Dental Care* 14(3): 111–116.

26 Saroglu, I., Sonmez, H. (2002). The prevalence of traumatic injuries treated in the pediatric clinic of Ankara University, Turkey, during 18 months. *Dental Traumatology* 18(6): 299–303.

27 Sheiham, A., Watt, R.G. (2000). The common risk factor approach: a rational basis for promoting oral health. *Community Dentistry and Oral Epidemiology* 28: 399–406.

28 Maughan, R.L., Murray, R. (2001). *Sports Drinks: Basic Science and Practical Aspects.* CRC Press, Boca Raton, London, New York, Washington DC.

29 Coombes, J.S., Hamilton, K.L. (2000). The effectiveness of commercially available sports drinks. *Sports Medicine.* 2000 29(3): 181–209.

30 Roy, B.D. (2008). Milk: the new sports drink?: a review. *Journal of the International Society of Sports Nutrition* 5(15). Doi: 10.1186/1550-2783-5-15.

31 How does milk affect athletic performance? *Cycling Weekly*, Oct 21, 2013.

32 Garner, D.P., McDivitt, E. (2009). Effects of mouthpiece use on airway openings and lactate levels in healthy college males. *Compendium of Continuing Education in Dentistry* 30 Spec No. 2:14–7.

33 Roettger, M. (2009). Performance enhancement and oral appliances. *Compendium of Continuing Education in Dentistry* 30 Spec No. 2:4–8

34 Duddy, F.A., Weissman, J., Lee, R.A., et al. (2012). Influence of different types of mouthguards on strength and performance of collegiate athletes: a controlled-randomised trial. *Dental Traumatology* 28: 263–267.

8

The Role of Nutrition in Sport: Current Sports Nutrition Advice
Gillian Horgan

8.1 Introduction

Nutrition is a key factor when considering sporting performance, and over recent years important developments in both the science and practice of sports nutrition have flourished. Whilst nutrition alone cannot make someone a better sportsperson, everyone is looking for an edge to improve their performance. Many people taking part in sport and exercise have improved their performance through the knowledge that energy consumed in the form of carbohydrate foods will increase muscle glycogen stores and carbohydrate oxidation, with such benefits as delayed onset of fatigue. There is now a wealth of knowledge on the need for optimal hydration for everyone who takes part in sport and exercise. This knowledge has helped individuals in their performance as well as informing organisers of sporting events about the need for the availability of suitable fluids; a huge industry has been created servicing this need. Individualised dietary strategies have helped to enhance performance and include optimising intakes, composition and timing of macronutrients, micronutrients, and fluids, and the judicious use of supplements.

Appropriately qualified, professional, registered sports dietitians and nutritionists can ensure that evidence-based research informs practice for all seeking advice.

The appreciation and importance of human muscle energy metabolism began in the mid-nineteenth century, when protein was considered the main fuel providing energy. Levine and colleagues in the 1920s observed low blood glucose levels of participants in the Boston marathon and linked these low levels to fatigue. Since these early experiments there has been steady progress in the understanding of the links between duration, intensity, timing, training, and nutrition. Studies from the 1960s demonstrated the importance of carbohydrate usage, the manipulation of fat as a substrate for energy, and the effect of limited stores of carbohydrates on performance. Dehydration and optimising fluid delivery through the use of sports drinks carried on through the 1980s and in 1991 the Medical Commission of the International Olympic Committee (IOC) published the first Consensus Statement on Nutrition and Athletic Performance. In 2003 and again in 2010 the IOC has conducted extensive reviews of the available research and knowledge on nutrition and nutritional intake in athletes, and produced consensus statements, which form the basis of advice given to athletes today [1].

More recently, different aspects of diet and sporting activity have been researched, including optimising nutrient timings, particularly of protein intake, to challenge metabolic adaptations and the use of the 'train low,

Sports Dentistry: Principles and Practice, First Edition. Edited by Peter D. Fine, Chris Louca and Albert Leung.
© 2019 John Wiley & Sons Ltd. Published 2019 by John Wiley & Sons Ltd.
Companion website: www.wiley.com/go/fine/sports_dentistry

compete high' protocol, which involves training with low levels of stored muscle glycogen, but allowing high carbohydrate availability during the competitive phase. Research into the potential performance advantages of using different dietary ergogenic aids (such as cherry juice and beetroot) has been explored. Recovery nutrition, nutrition to promote immune function and gut health in athletes, and building muscle through diet, as well as weight management are all current issues that are of interest to the athlete. Nowadays advice is from evidence-based sports nutrition guidelines, which are based on sound scientific research. The quantity, quality, timing, and type of food and drink consumed are of utmost importance to enhance the metabolic adaptations to training and recovery, so athletes can reach their potential, as injury and illness-free as possible.

A variety of foods containing macronutrients (carbohydrates, proteins, and fats) to provide energy, and micronutrients (vitamins and minerals) to optimise health, as well as sufficient and appropriate fluids, are all essential for performance. Habitual and well-timed carbohydrate intake before, during and after exercise is necessary for optimal training and performance. Protein recommendations, whilst already more than sufficient for the majority of the UK population, are slightly higher for those wanting to achieve an increase in strength and power, and those who partake in frequent endurance exercise. Fat intakes should be from foods that contain unsaturated fatty acids, giving optimal intakes of essential fatty acids and fat-soluble vitamins, whilst maintaining energy balance. Micronutrients can be consumed through the regular consumption of a variety of foods, in particular fruits and vegetables. Further research is needed to establish if higher amounts are needed for the sporting population. Finally, some supplements, including sports foods may be of benefit in certain situations for certain individuals, but need to be carefully considered.

When considering the diet for an athlete, one of the first questions to ask is whether the athlete is someone who is aiming for the Olympics or World Championships, or someone who is a motivated amateur and just wants to survive running 26.2 miles of a marathon, or play tennis, rugby, football, cricket at the weekend. Or is it someone who likes to take part in challenging events on occasions such as 'marathon des sables', 'tough mudder', or similar? Whether the goal is a gold medal or whether it is to lose weight, to generally get fitter and healthier, or because a doctor suggested it... the advice has to be tailored to fit the individual. However, there are some general recommendations on energy and macro- and micronutrient intake, as well as hydration strategies that are useful for all.

Underpinning all the advice about eating for exercise and sport is the principle that the body needs good nutrition, whatever is being asked of it and a good place to start is Public Health England's *Eatwell Guide* [2]. Food provides the body with the energy and nutrients it needs for growth, development and maintenance to meet daily lifestyle requirements for health and wellbeing.

The body's energy supply comes from the macronutrients in our diet – carbohydrate, protein, fat (alcohol also provides energy) (see Table 8.1). Food and drinks contain differing amounts of these nutrients and when they are digested and absorbed contribute to the overall energy (kilocalorie) content of the diet.

Table 8.1 Energy sources from food and drinks.

Sources of Energy	Kilocalories/g
Carbohydrate	3.75
Protein	4
Fat	9
Alcohol	7

8.2 What is the Optimal Diet for an Athlete? Is it Different for the Recreational Exerciser?

8.2.1 Energy

- Correct energy intake – not too much, not too little – is needed for health and to perform well.
- Stable body weight is a crude, but easy method to monitor energy requirements.
- Energy comes from a mix of fuels – carbohydrates and fats in particular.
- Low energy availability can cause problems, especially for young female exercisers.

The first priority is to consider baseline energy requirements – whatever level and whatever intensity and duration of exercise – the body needs energy in the form of food and drink.

Mostly, energy intake requirements are increased to compensate for the energy used during exercise. Some of the energy consumed as food and drink is used straight away, but most is stored until it is needed later on. The body uses different energy systems for different types of activity (ATP-CP/aerobic and anaerobic), all provided by the carbohydrates, fats, and proteins in the diet, with the aim of providing adenosine triphosphate (ATP) for energy production (Figure 8.1). All the energy

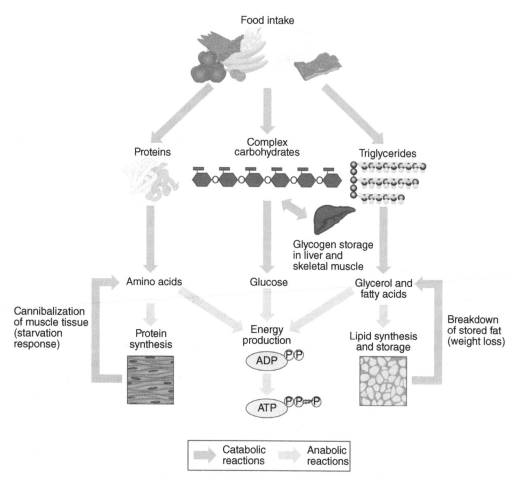

Figure 8.1 Energy supply systems.

required during muscular contraction is powered by energy released when ATP is converted into adenosine diphosphate (ADP). Only a small amount of ATP is available in muscle cells and must be maintained, therefore ATP will only support a few seconds' worth of exercise.

A second source of energy is creatine phosphate (CP), also found in muscle cells. Transfer of a phosphate group from CP to ADP resynthesises ATP in the presence of the enzyme creatine kinase. Energy can be supplied at a very fast rate through these processes, but the capacity is limited. For prolonged exercise, glycogen (carbohydrate stored in muscles) is used. Although storage in the muscles (and a small amount in the liver) is reasonably limited and variable, energy can be made available through a series of reactions (Figure 8.1). All fuels (carbohydrate, fat, and protein) can be used by muscle cells to produce energy during exercise, but for fat the rate at which energy can be produced is much less than can be achieved through the oxidation of carbohydrate. The advantage of using fat as a fuel lies in its storage capacity, as the body can store large amounts. A very small amount of protein is available as an energy source during exercise.

The amount of energy needed varies from individual to individual and the amount of energy expended varies likewise. The correct energy requirements of individual athletes, particularly at the elite level, needs to be carefully calculated by a skilled and experienced nutritionist. The energy reference values defined in the Scientific Advisory Committee on Nutrition (SACN) [3] report are derived for infants, children, and adults in relation to body weights, likely to be consistent with long-term good health. For serious exercisers and athletes, there is a need to consume enough energy to maintain appropriate weight and body composition while training for a sport.

For someone competing at higher levels there are prediction equations in the literature which predict basal metabolic rate (BMR) and an activity component or physical activity level (PAL), and energy intake can be calculated from body size, age, and gender.

For those not competing at these levels who do not need accurate measurements, a simple step to ensure sufficient energy intake includes a stable body weight (although not necessarily an accurate marker). However, if weight is in the right range and stable for a period of time and the person is consuming a variety of nutritious foods, this indicates energy intake is sufficient. Trends in weight change up or down over a week or more indicates an imbalance between energy consumed and energy expended. Skinfold thickness measures using callipers or a BodPod* can give a more accurate measure of body composition and energy needs. For most people, a stable weight is sufficient.

Some athletes who compete in endurance and aesthetic or weight-category sports frequently restrict their energy intake. Literature shows that these athletes, and particularly female athletes, reduce their intake by up to 30% of that recommended, affecting energy availability. Energy availability is defined by the total energy intake minus the energy used in daily activity and exercise, and if insufficient means there is lack of available energy for health, growth, and development, with implications on reproductive and immune systems (see section on eating disorders)

8.2.2 Carbohydrates

- Carbohydrates are the most important foods for fuelling the body during exercise.
- Focus on carbohydrate rich foods at mealtimes.
- Body stores are limited so need restocking (if they have been used up by exercise).
- Carbohydrate foods designed for sporting purposes have implications for oral health.

---

* The Bod Pod is an air displacement plethysmograph, which uses whole-body densitometry to determine body composition (fat and fat-free mass). The system is safe, non-invasive, and has excellent test-to-test repeatability.

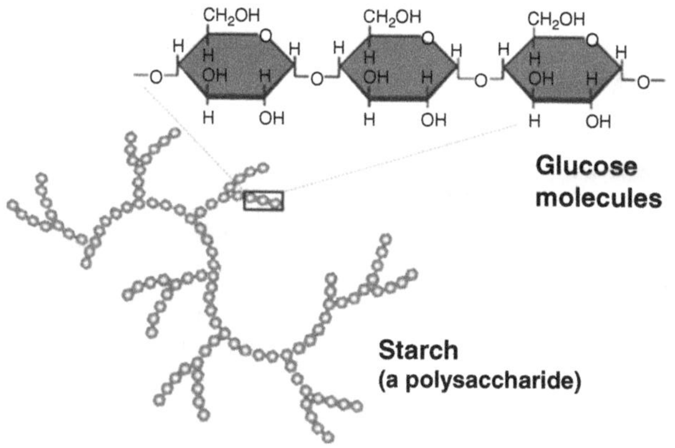

Polysaccharides

Glucose
molecules

Starch
(a polysaccharide)

Figure 8.2 Basic units of carbohydrates.

Carbohydrates are sources of metabolic fuels and energy. Many foods are rich in carbohydrates, including cereals, potatoes, rice, pasta, and other grains such as quinoa, barley, and wheat. These foods are also high in B vitamins needed for efficient energy production. Many fruits and some vegetables are high in carbohydrates, as well as being high in the natural antioxidant vitamin C, which helps maintain a healthy immune system. The regular need to replace carbohydrate in elite athletes results in the mouth being constantly bathed in sugars, which can lead to deterioration of dental health, together with poor oral hygiene, resulting in dental caries and the need for ongoing dental treatment.

Carbohydrates are diverse molecules and are composed of different sugars, oligosaccharides, and polysaccharides (Figure 8.2).

Glucose is sometimes found naturally in foods, but is usually derived from the digestion of other carbohydrates. Fructose is found naturally in honey and most fruits, and from the digestion of sucrose (sucrose is made up of glucose + fructose). Galactose can be found naturally in food, but mostly stems from the digestion of lactose, found mainly in milk and dairy foods (lactose is made up of glucose and galactose). High fructose corn syrup (HFCS) is a popular food-sweetening additive (a fructose–glucose liquid sweetener) and is often more than 50–60% fructose. The food industry use HFCS over sucrose in foods and drinks because of its sweetness, stability, and functionality. Naturally occurring sugars in foods such as honey, fruits, and milk and milk products, as well as sugars added during the processing of foods and drinks, such as HFCS, malt, and dextrose, are introduced to the mouth, where they start digestion.

Carbohydrates can be classified into different groups (see Table 8.2).

The chemical nature of carbohydrates and their molecular structure within the foods of which they are part, determine their digestive fate. Once taken into the oral cavity, digestion of carbohydrates begins in the mouth. Salivary α-amylase is the major enzyme secreted by the salivary glands, which hydrolyses the bonds in the polysaccharide carbohydrates amylose and amylopectin to release the simple sugars maltose, maltotriose and dextrins. These may be fermented by the oral microflora, causing a drop in dental plaque pH and potential subsequent caries formation. Not all carbohydrates are equally cariogenic. Those that are readily fermented by bacteria in the mouth are those sugars commonly found in food such as glucose, sucrose, fructose, and maltose. Those that are less cariogenic are lactose, galactose, and starches. Sugar alcohols such as xylitol are non-cariogenic. To lower the risk of dental

Table 8.2 Classes, sources, and examples of different carbohydrates and artificial sweeteners.

Groups of carbohydrates	Typical dietary source	Example
• Free sugars (monosaccharides)		Glucose Fructose Galactose
• Disaccharides		Sucrose Lactose Maltose
• Sugar alcohols		Xylitol Sorbitol
• Short-chain carbohydrates (oligosaccharides)		Inulin
• Starch (polysaccharides) • Rapidly digestible starch (RDS) • Slowly digestible starch (SDS)		Starches
• Resistant starch		
• Non-starch polysaccharides (NSPs) • Cell-wall NSPs in unrefined plant foods (dietary fibre)		
• Other NSPs, e.g. pectin		

Sweeteners	Relative sweetness compared to table sugar (sucrose)
• Natural Sweetener	
Stevia	300
• Artificial Sweetener	
Aspartame	180
Saccharin	300
Sucrolose	600
Acesulfame - K	180
• Caloric sweetener	
High fructose corn syrup (HFCS)	1.2–1.6

caries, eating sugars with meals and including something that contains phosphates (helps prevent demineralisation), such as cheese, helps.

The preferred energy fuel for muscular contraction is carbohydrates – this is the only fuel that can support moderate- to high-intensity exercise. Carbohydrates maintain blood glucose during exercise and replace muscle glycogen after exercise. However, the body can only store a limited amount of carbohydrate in the form of liver and muscle glycogen, which generally can only fuel someone for a couple of hours. Carbohydrates (glucose) are also used as an source of energy to fuel the brain.

8.2.2.1   Low Levels of Glycogen Result in Early Fatigue

It is clear from extensive research that those who regularly exercise to compete need daily total dietary carbohydrates targets, and general recommendations should be expressed as grams of carbohydrate per kilogram of an athlete's body weight rather than a percentage of their total energy intake, to take account of differing body sizes. Guidelines are often based on daily exercise patterns and durations (Table 8.3).

These guidelines have to be carefully interpreted, taking into account someone's overall needs for energy, their training programme and requirements for growth and development in the case of children and adolescents. A small, young female swimmer training twice a day and spending hours at the pool would, according to this chart require in the region of 8–12 g/kg body weight. This is unlikely as there are down periods of low intensity or coach education where there is no activity and so 'common sense' equations and knowledge of the sport have to be factored in.

8.2.2.2   During Exercise

If the activity is prolonged, as in endurance exercise (long distance running and cycling for instance), fuel can be consumed during the exercise to help provide extra 'top-up' energy. This helps maintain blood glucose concentrations, high rates of carbohydrate utilisation, and spares the stored muscle glycogen for later use. For endurance events lasting more than 90–120 minutes the advice is to consume some carbohydrate during exercise. For team or multi-sprint sports lasting more than 60 minutes (football, rugby) there is evidence that taking on some carbohydrate may also be helpful. Sports drinks, gels, bars, and jelly beans have all been used to supply the carbohydrate during exercise, and studies have shown an equal ability to affect performance positively [5]. However, since there is often a need to stay hydrated, an athlete needs to think about fluids as well as fuel, and sports drinks serve both purposes, which is why they are so popular.

What is of importance is the amount of carbohydrate and the types of sugars that make up the carbohydrate. Studies have shown that the maximum oxidation rate for glucose-based drinks is 60 g/h. If one consumes more than this, the drink remains in the stomach longer, potentially causing gastrointestinal distress. However, there are a variety of drinks/gels on the market which contain combinations of different sugars (glucose and fructose). Once consumed, carbohydrates need to be absorbed into the intestine. Different sugars use different intestinal transporters to achieve this. Glucose uses SGLT1

Table 8.3   2010 Guidelines/Categories – daily needs for fuel and recovery (consider total energy needs, specific training needs, feedback from training) [4].

Activity	g carbohydrate/kg body weight/day
Low-intensity or skill-based activities	3–5
Moderate exercise programme, i.e. 1 h per day	5–7
Endurance programme, i.e. 1–3 h per day Moderate–high intensity	6–10
Extreme commitment, i.e. > 4–5 h per day Moderate–high intensity	8–12

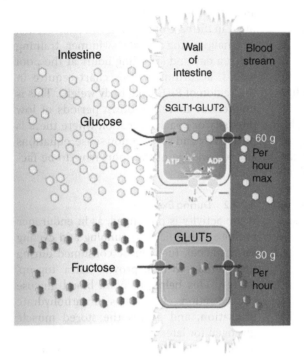

Figure 8.3 Use of different multiple transportable carbohydrates (glucose and fructose) results in greater fluid and carbohydrate delivery compared to glucose alone (Taken from: https://highfive.co.uk/high5-faster-and-further/21-fructose-and-caffeine/)

transporter and fructose, GLUT5. When the glucose SGLT1 transporter becomes saturated no more can be absorbed – or transported to the working muscle. By using a different sugar and transporter, additional carbohydrate (fructose) can be delivered to the muscle, thereby making more energy available for use. These are called multiple transportable carbohydrates (Figure 8.3). Recent studies have shown improvement in performance of long distance runners and cyclists using these products [6].

Recent studies looking at endurance activities lasting less than one hour have reported positive effects on performance by using carbohydrate mouth rinses, whereby sugar solutions are swilled around in the mouth, but not swallowed [7]. This has implications for dental health as it allows contact between sugars and the tooth enamel. (See Section 8.3.1 on sports drinks for further information).

8.2.3 Protein

Protein intake in athletes have been recommended in order to support metabolic adaptation, repair, and remodelling. Those specifically wanting to increase muscle mass and strength need to stimulate muscle protein synthesis (MPS) through resistance training and protein intake providing between 1.2 and 2.0 g/kg/day. Higher intakes may be indicated for short periods during intensified training or when reducing energy intake. Daily protein intake goals should be met with a meal plan providing a regular spread of moderate amounts of high-quality protein (15–25 g/meal or snack) across the day and following strenuous training sessions. These amounts can be met through consuming meat, fish, eggs, dairy products, cereals, and some vegetables, which are widely available, therefore protein supplements such as whey powders and amino acid mixes are not necessary.

Guidelines are based around meeting optimal energy and other nutrient requirements [8].

These recommendations also depend on the training status of the athlete; trained athletes would require lower levels and those starting out training to increase muscle mass would require higher levels. Higher doses of more than 40 g protein at any meal or snack have not yet been shown to further boost MPS and may only be advised for the largest athletes, or during weight loss.

8.2.4 Recovery

As the body undergoes repair and adaptation after exercise and gets ready for the next exercise bout, intakes of carbohydrate and protein are necessary. Studies show there is a slightly higher rate of glycogen restoration in the couple of hours after exercise. However, for most exercisers the important factor is getting access to a carbohydrate and protein supply. If, as for most people, there is more than eight hours before the next workout or exercise session, there is not such a great necessity in replacing the nutrients immediately. If time between exercise bouts is shorter, for instance playing in a tournament such as rugby 7s or netball then they would be advised to have a supply of suitable recovery snacks to hand to optimise this slightly higher rate of glycogen restoration. The target is usually between 1 and 1.2g carbohydrate per kilogram body weight and around 20g of protein. Chronic training studies have shown that the consumption of milk-based protein after resistance exercise is effective in increasing muscle strength and favourable changes in body composition [9].

Practical advice would be to consume foods which contain all the above nutrients, as well as fluid such as milk or milkshakes, which are convenient. However, other snacks such as meat, chicken, or tuna sandwiches are helpful; relying on protein supplements at this point is unnecessary.

8.2.5 Fats

Fat is a necessary component of a healthy diet, providing energy, fat-soluble vitamins, and essential fatty acids. The UK dietary guidelines have made recommendations that energy from saturated fats should be limited to 10% of the total intake and the diet should include sources of omega-3 fats and other unsaturated fats. Sources of these include: nuts, seeds, and oily fish, such as salmon, mackerel, sardines, and fresh tuna, as well as spreads and oils that are produced using predominantly unsaturated fat sources. Intake of fat by athletes should be in accordance with these guidelines and should be individualised based on training level and body composition goals.

Fat is the other major fuel contributing to oxidative metabolism during prolonged exercise. Fat that is stored in adipose tissue can be made available more readily through exercise-induced endurance training, which increases sources of energy available for oxidation. Dietary strategies such as fat loading, high-fat diets, and fasting have all been used to demonstrate an enhancement of exercise capacity at moderate intensity levels. There seems to be a down-regulation of carbohydrate, which spares the limited stores of carbohydrate, potentially allowing muscle to use more fat as a source of energy. However, the debate as to whether to advise enhancing exercise performance through dietary fat manipulation is still ongoing, and competitive athletes would be unwise to follow these theories at the moment. Athletes who constantly restrict their fat intake to lose body fat and weight should be advised to still continue to include some unsaturated fats in their diet.

8.2.6 Vitamins, Minerals, and Trace Elements

Micronutrients play an important role in energy production, synthesis of haemoglobin, bone health, an efficient immune system, and defence against oxidative damage, which occurs more rapidly when exercising vigorously. Although exercise may increase the turnover and loss of micronutrients from the body, there is no specific sports nutrition recommendation to increase them, although many active people do take vitamin/mineral supplements. It is generally accepted that athletes need an adequate intake (at least to the level of the reference nutrient intake – RNI), and these are best consumed as part of a good eating plan. This translates into a variety of foods, in particular a good supply of fruits and vegetables.

There are some athletes who would benefit from a micronutrient supplement. Supplementation of certain single vitamins or minerals is usually only appropriate to correct a clinical deficiency such as vitamin D, calcium, and iron. There are those exercisers who frequently restrict energy intake, rely on extreme weight-loss practices, eliminate one or more food groups from their diet, or consume poorly chosen diets who would benefit from a daily multivitamin/mineral supplement to correct these low levels, but this alone will not improve performance, only correct a nutritionally poor diet.

8.2.7 Micronutrients of Interest

8.2.7.1 Calcium

Most people understand the connection between calcium, bones, and teeth. Calcium is also required for muscle contraction and normal blood clotting. However, the vast majority of people get enough calcium in their normal diets. Together with Vitamin D, calcium is needed to alleviate the risk of low bone mineral density and potential stress fractures. Female athletes are particularly prone to low bone mineral density, especially if they avoid calcium-containing dairy foods due to an ill-planned weight-reducing diet.

8.2.7.2 Vitamin D

Vitamin D is required for adequate calcium absorption and bone health. A growing number of studies have documented the relationship between vitamin D status and sport: injury prevention, rehabilitation, improved neuromuscular function, increased type II muscle fibre size, reduced inflammation, decreased risk of stress fracture, and acute respiratory illness. Recently, Public Health England (PHE) has recommended that adults and children over the age of one should have 10 micrograms of vitamin D every day. The advice is based on the report from the government's Scientific Advisory Committee on Nutrition (SACN), following its review of the evidence on vitamin D and health [10]. As foods containing vitamin D are quite sparse – oily fish, fortified margarines, some breakfast cereals, and fortified milks, the advice, especially for those who live in northern latitudes or who train primarily indoors all year (gymnasts, swimmers, ice skaters) is to take a daily supplement. Seek further advice on anti-doping for tested athletes.

8.2.7.3 Iron

Iron deficiency is bad news for general life, let alone for a serious exerciser. Iron depletion is the most common nutrient deficiency seen in female athletes, especially if they are vegetarian or vegan (due to poor iron bioavailability from the foods they consume). Most become aware when they feel unusually tired on an ongoing basis. Utter fatigue can diminish even the most committed exerciser from taking part in exercise.

Iron is required for the formation of haemoglobin and myoglobin. Oxygen carrying capacity is essential for endurance exercise.

8.2.7.4 Antioxidants

The end result of muscular contractions is free radical production (pro-oxidants) and potential muscle cell damage. Antioxidants contained in foods can help to mitigate against this damage although there is limited evidence. Common antioxidants are glutathione, vitamins C and E, β-carotene, and selenium, found in a variety of fruits and vegetables.

Athletes at greatest risk for poor antioxidant intakes are those who restrict energy intake, follow a chronic low-fat diet, or limit dietary intake of fruits, vegetables and whole grains.

8.3 Hydration

Fluids and electrolytes are regularly consumed to maintain optimal hydration before, during, and after exercise. This is needed for physiological functions such as thermoregulation and the transport of nutrients around the body. Hypohydration impairs performance and increases the risk of heat illness during exercise.

There is still much debate about advice given on fluid intake. The American College of Sports Medicine's (ACSM) Position Paper on Exercise and Fluid Replacement provides a comprehensive review of the research and recommendations for maintaining hydration before, during, and after exercise [11].

General consensus statements have been published, which state that:

- Hypohydration can negatively affect physical and mental preparation and performance.
- More than 2% loss of body weight through sweating can impair aerobic performance, particularly in warm climates.
- Tests of strength and power are largely unaffected by dehydration of up to about 2–4% of body mass.
- However, weight loss of 1–2% seems not to affect aerobic performance in temperate climes (20–21 °C) if the activity lasts less than 90 minutes.
- There seems to be little effect on performance in anaerobic activities of moderate hypohydration and hyperthermia.
- More than 3% body weight loss combined with heat stress may influence cognitive function, mood, and mental readiness.
- Dehydration can occur in cold climates due to respiratory losses and insulated warm clothing increasing sweat loss. In cold climates, cold drinks are often not readily consumed and not wanting to take off layers of clothing to urinate often precludes much drinking of fluids.
- Higher fluid losses may occur when exercising at altitude compared to sea level training.

To re-establish euhydration both water and electrolytes (in particular sodium) can be consumed through subsequent food and drinks if there is no time urgency in replacing losses. If recovery is more important, such as when replacement is needed to normalise water balance within 24 hours to prepare for later exercise bouts or when hypohydration is severe (<5%), a personalised hydration strategy is needed.

Measuring hydration status is governed by the need for sensitivity and accuracy,

Pee chart

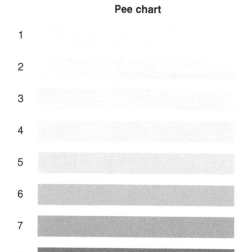

1

2

3

4

5

6

7

8

Your target is to make sure that your pee is the same colour as numbers 1, 2 or 3.

Figure 8.4 Urine colour chart.

together with technical expertise, costs, and time involvement. Overall, practicality of monitoring hydration status is needed. Markers such as acute changes in body weight during exercise, due to sweating, are relatively easy to measure and can indicate the degree of dehydration, as long as any food and drink consumed during the activity is accounted for. Urinary indices such as volume and colour can also be used as hydration markers. Urine colour charts are widely used as a field measure of hydration, but are subject to individual interpretation (Figure 8.4) Urinary specific gravity and osmolality can also be used to approximate hydration status by measuring the concentration of the solutes in urine. When assessed from a midstream collection of the first morning urine sample, a urinary specific gravity of <1.020 to <1.025 is generally indicative of euhydration. Urinary osmolality reflects hypohydration when >900 mOsmol/kg, while euhydration is considered to be <700 mOsmol/kg (Figure 8.5). Invasive techniques using blood can be used, but have obvious disadvantages, especially in the field setting where sporting activities take place.

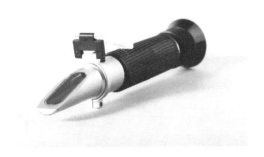

Figure 8.5 Monitoring fluid status.

8.3.1 Sports Drinks

During high-intensity exercise, prolonged endurance activities, and intermittent team sports, both carbohydrate and fluid reserves become depleted; they can be replenished by consuming a sports drink. Sports drinks can also be used to recover energy and fluid reserves quickly after a weigh in and before competition in weight-category sports. The main carbohydrates used in sports drinks are glucose, fructose, sucrose, and malto-dextrins, also known as glucose polymers. It is well known that increasing the concentration of carbohydrate, and thereby producing an increase in osmolality in a drink, will impair gastric emptying and hence the absorption of fluid. The use of glucose polymers in sports drinks has allowed for provision of more carbohydrate without a resultant increase in osmolality or unpalatability.

The optimum concentration for a sports drink is dependent on the requirement of the individual. Providing high carbohydrate levels in a sports drink will deliver more available energy to the working muscle, but will delay gastric emptying, thereby reducing the amount of fluid that is available for absorption. These drinks provide carbohydrates in the region of <8 g/100 ml fluid and are termed *hypertonic*. In warm climates where sweat losses are reasonably high, these drinks may actually increase the danger of dehydration. In climates when sweat rates are low, but energy requirements are high these are the drinks of choice.

Isotonic sports drinks are the most commonly used sports drinks. These drinks are formulated so the osmolality of the drink is as similar to body fluids as possible, to promote gastric emptying rates and absorption. Carbohydrate concentrations of isotonic drinks are generally in the region of 4–8 g/100 ml fluid.

For most rapid rehydration *hypotonic* drinks are advised, especially in hot climates where fluid delivery is the most important element, rather than the need to fuel the muscles. Hypotonic drinks usually contain 2–4 g carbohydrate/100 ml fluid.

Sodium chloride or sodium citrate are added to sports drinks to help stimulate the uptake of sugar and water into the small intestine and maintain extracellular fluid volume. Sports drinks generally contain between 10–30 mmol/l of sodium chloride/citrate. Specialised sports drinks are formulated with higher levels, especially helpful for activities in hot climates, but the disadvantage of high sodium levels is that the drink becomes unpalatable, so often a compromise has to be reached. Sports drinks can also include 3–5 mmol/l of potassium.

Sugar-sweetened beverages (SSBs) are associated with dental caries [12]. Sports drinks that are essentially SSBs are a concern for oral health for a number of reasons. They are acidic (around pH 2.4–4.5), with such ingredients as malic acid or citric acid included in their formulation. This can be damaging to the tooth enamel, leading to dental erosion. Sports drinks are relatively low in carbohydrate (sugar) to assist the active person in provision of energy for the working muscles, but tend to be sipped frequently during exercise (rather than consuming all at once). Frequent sipping increases the contact time that teeth are exposed to the acidic environment. If carbohydrate mouth rinse practices are adopted, this can also negatively affect dental health.

The saliva in the mouth helps to neutralise the acids, providing calcium and phosphate to remineralise tooth enamel. However, dehydration causes the mouth to become dry, reducing salivary flow, and also increasing the potential for tooth erosion and decay.

8.4 Supplements

Supplement refers to something that should supplement the normal diet, not replace it. The use of dietary supplements is widespread among athletes. In light of this, a pragmatic approach to advice regarding supplements and sports foods/drinks is needed. Some can contribute to a well-designed sports eating plan and can directly or indirectly enhance performance. Supplements such as caffeine, sports drinks/gels /creatine have been shown to be effective when taken as part of a well-chosen eating plan for some athletes (Table 8.4). Athletes should be advised by registered sports dietitians/nutritionists on whether or not supplements will benefit them individually.

However, there are some sports products that may have an influence on dental health. Sports drinks have already been considered. Sports gels and bars are highly concentrated forms of carbohydrate (sugars) that have the potential to coat teeth after consumption. Gels usually contain between 25 and 40 g carbohydrate per gel or bar, and are often used during long-distance endurance events, such as marathon running or cycling. To meet fluid needs they are often consumed with water or other fluids. Although water may help to flush some of the solution away, damage through dental erosion can still occur.

8.5 Gastro-intestinal Complaints Related to Exercise

Exercise causes changes to circulation, ischaemia, and increased mucosal permeability, blood flow to the gastrointestinal tract can reduce by 80%, and subsequent nausea,

vomiting, abdominal pain, and diarrhoea can follow [13].

Advice includes:

- Avoid high-fibre foods on the day or even days before competition
- Avoid aspirin and NSAIDs such as ibuprofen. Both have commonly been shown to increase intestinal permeability and may increase the incidence of gastrointestinal complaints.
- Avoid high-fructose foods (in particular drinks that are exclusively fructose).
- Avoid dehydration, which can exacerbate gastrointestinal symptoms.
- Ingest carbohydrates with sufficient water or choose drinks with lower carbohydrate concentrations.
- Consume a low-fibre diet 24–28 hours before an event.
- Practise new nutrition strategies before race day.

8.6 Eating Disorders in Sport

Researchers reported on the incidence of eating disorders in a group of 1620 elite competitors [14]. Research supported earlier findings that athletes are at higher risk of having an eating disorder than non-athletic controls. Risk is highest in sports where weight is a factor in performance or there is an aesthetic aspect. These sports include endurance sports (such as distance running), weight-class sports (such as wrestling), and aesthetic sports such as gymnastics and anti-gravity sports (such as ski-jumping).

An eating disorder is a health problem in which an unusual or disordered eating pattern is central, and associated with emotional and physical harm. There are different presentations of eating disorders: disordered eating, anorexia nervosa, bulimia nervosa, atypical (or sub-clinical) disorders, such as anorexia athletica and the female athlete triad, relative energy deficiency in sport (RED-S), eating disorders not otherwise

Table 8.4 Supplements that can be considered within a well-balanced food plan.

Nutrient	Supplement	Foods
Iron Periods of rapid growth (the adolescent athlete), training at high altitudes, menstrual blood loss, foot-strike haemolysis or injury can negatively influence iron status. Athletes who are at greatest risk, such as distance runners, females in aesthetic sports, vegetarian athletes, or regular blood donors, should be screened regularly and aim for an iron intake greater than their RNI (i.e. >14.8 mg for women and >8.7 mg for men).	Ferrous sulfate supplement could help. Iron supplementation not only improves blood biochemical measures and iron status, but also increases work capacity, as evidenced by increasing oxygen uptake, reducing heart rate, and decreasing lactate concentration during exercise. Recent findings provide additional support for improved performance (i.e. less skeletal muscle fatigue) when iron supplementation was prescribed.	Red meat, liver and offal, fortified breakfast cereals, eggs, wholegrain bread, dark green leafy vegetables, pulses, dried fruit, nuts and seeds. Animal sources of iron have greater bioavailability. Take with vitamin C to promote absorption, e.g. blackcurrants or other berries with porridge for breakfast.
Calcium and Vitamin D Low calcium intakes are associated with restricted energy intake, disordered eating, and/or the specific avoidance of dairy products or other calcium-rich foods Athletes who primarily train indoors or train in the early morning and evening when ultraviolet B light (UVB) levels are low, have a dark complexion, high body fat content, or block UVB exposure with clothing, equipment, and suntan lotions increase the risk of vitamin D deficiency.	Calcium supplementation should be determined after a thorough assessment of usual dietary intake.	Calcium-containing foods include milk and milk products, such as cheese and yoghurts, small fish containing soft bones, such as sardines, fortified white flour products, such as bread and cereals, and dark green leafy vegetables. Vitamin D-containing foods include oily fish, such as salmon, sardines, herring, mackerel, and fresh tuna, red meat, liver, egg yolks, and fortified foods such as fat spreads and some breakfast cereals.

specified (EDNOS). For someone who is focused on sport and exercise they may be seen as 'unusual eaters', where there is a meticulous attention to diet and weight, they are very goal-orientated, and their aim is performance enhancement. The emphasis is on adequate intake rather than restriction (what is needed rather than what is forbidden) and this is likely to 'normalise' when sport ceases. For someone who is leaning towards more disordered eating pattern it is likely that they will use pathogenic weight control measures such as laxatives, diuretics, enemas, diet pills, stimulants, and/or self-induced vomiting. Often there is a history of 'excessive' exercise (e.g. secret or extra training) as well as extreme, restrictive, or 'faddy' diets.

8.6.1 Special Concerns for the Female Athlete

The female athlete triad is a term used when the following conditions exist together: disordered eating + amenorrhoea + osteoporosis [15]. More recently, the term relative energy deficiency in sport (RED-S) has been used, which includes males as well as females. The syndrome of RED-S refers to impaired physiological functioning caused by relative energy deficiency, and includes, but is not limited to impairments of metabolic rate, menstrual function, bone health, immunity, protein synthesis, and cardiovascular health. RED-S is termed 'low energy availability', where an individual's dietary energy intake is insufficient to support the energy expenditure required for health, function, and daily living, once the cost of exercise and sporting activities is taken into account.

8.6.1.1 Effect on Health
The effect of RED-S on health is shown in Figure 8.6.

8.6.1.2 Effect on Performance
The potential effects of RED-S on performance are shown in Figure 8.7.

8.6.1.3 The RED-S CAT
The RED-S CAT is based on the IOC Consensus Statement [17] and is a clinical

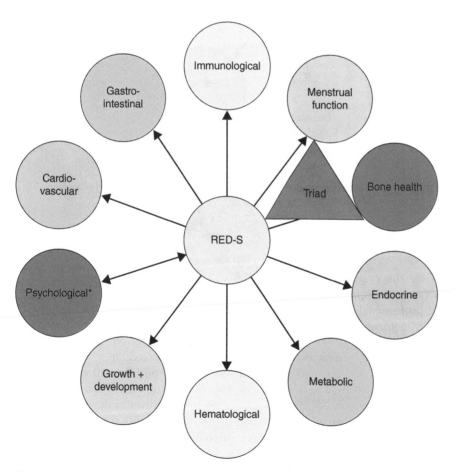

Figure 8.6 Health consequences of relative energy deficiency in sport (RED-S) showing an expanded concept of the female athlete triad to acknowledge a wider range of outcomes and the application to male athletes (*Psychological consequences can either precede RED-S or be the result of RED-S). (Adapted from Constantini [16].)

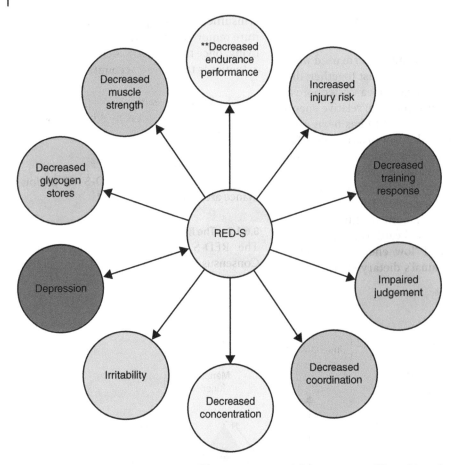

Figure 8.7 Potential performance effects of relative energy deficiency in sport (** aerobic and anaerobic performance). (Adapted from Constantini [16].)

assessment tool for the evaluation of athletes/active play decisions. It is designed for use by a medical professional in the clinical evaluation and management of athletes with this syndrome.

Treatment of low energy availability should involve an increase in energy intake, reduction in exercise or a combination of both. The only strategy to be researched is the addition of an energy-rich supplement to the normal diet plus the introduction of a rest day. A practical approach would be to increase the daily energy intake by 300–600 kcal/day and address the sub-optimal training practices and food-related stress.

8.7 The Future

Over the last decade there have been many publications, including consensus statements and recommendations on sports nutrition advice, as well as accreditation and qualifications awarded to sports nutrition practitioners. This flourishing area of sports nutrition continues to strengthen as the weight of evidence from good-quality research increases. Nutritional advice and goals are not static and need to be reviewed constantly, in line with training and competition programmes that are personalised to each athlete, their event, their goals, their practical challenges, and their food preferences.

More recent work has focused on the manipulation of nutrients such as:

- *Training low*: whereby limited or no carbohydrate is consumed between two exercise sessions. The first session will lower the available carbohydrate stores so that the second training session is performed in a low glycogen state. This is thought to increase the expression of relevant genes that stimulate fat catabolism and mitochondrial biogenesis, and as such improves oxidative capacity. In short, training in a muscle glycogen-depleted state increases the ability to oxidise fat and use it as a fuel, which for long endurance events means that there is a delay in fatigue and potential improvement in performance
- *Training the gut*: to increase gastric emptying and avoid stomach distress. Problems with stomach distress are very common among endurance runners. It is likely that this is due to reduced blood flow to the intestine during prolonged exercise. Training the gut could help the delivery of nutrients such as carbohydrate.
- If symptoms are not caused by exercise and a GP diagnosis of irritable bowel syndrome is thought to be the cause, then referral to a FODMAP-trained dietitian could be trialed. FODMAP foods (detailed below) are carbohydrates that are poorly absorbed by the gut. The intestinal bacteria in the gut react to certain foods and cause abdominal pain, gas, bloating, diarrhoea, and/or constipation [18].

F = Fermentable (produce gas)
O = Oligosaccharides (fructo- and galacto-oligosaccharides)
D = Disaccharides (lactose)
M = Monosaccharides (fructose)
A = And

P = Polyols (sorbitol and mannitol)

This diet should be supervised by a FODMAP-trained experienced dietitian.

8.8 Summary

For serious athletes there is a need for a long-term, comprehensively planned approach to their dietary intake, which takes into account their training and competition commitments. This cannot be done with just the athlete and the nutritionist, the coach, team members and other significant people involved with that athlete need to be on board.

For the weekend exercisers whose nutrition is still important in order to compete/finish/increase fitness or change body composition there needs to be an understanding of good nutritional practices and strategies that work for them. There is a growing trend for individualised dietary plans linked to periodisation training.

There are emerging concepts such as training with low carbohydrate or training whilst fasting to initiate adaptation to training. Whatever is the new approach there is still a need for balanced, healthy nutrition overall, taking care that all micronutrients are included and not overtaken by the desire to eat more carbohydrate and protein foods. Hydration practices should be personalised and simply monitored. Advice on supplements needs to be rational: is there a medical need for them or is there is sufficient robust evidence that they are safe and will help performance. Like training, getting the diet right takes practice, practice, practice, but ultimately food choices should be healthy, balanced, and enjoyable.

References

1 Maughan, R.J., Shirreffs, S.M. (2011). *Proceedings of the IOC Consensus Conference on Nutrition in Sport, 25–27 October 2010*, International Olympic Committee, Lausanne, Switzerland.

2 Public Health England's Eatwell Guide (2018). www.bda.uk.com/foodfacts/food_fact_sheet_information_sources/healthyeatinginfo (accessed April 2018).

3 Scientific Advisory Committee on Nutrition (2011). *Dietary Reference Values for Energy.* TSO, London.

4 Thomas, D.T., Erdman, K.A., Burke, L.M. (2016). Position of the academy of nutrition and dietetics, dietitians of Canada, and the American college of sports medicine: nutrition and athletic performance. *Journal of the Academy of Nutrition and Dietetics* 116(3): 501–528.

5 Jeukendrup, A. (2004). Carbohydrate intake during exercise and performance. *Nutrition*, 20(7–8): 669–677.

6 Currell, K., Jeukendrup, A.E. (2008). Superior endurance performance with ingestion of multiple transportable carbohydrates. *Medicine and Science in Sports and Exercise* 40(2): 275–281.

7 Ataide-Silva, T., de Souza, M.E.D.C.A., de Amorim, J.F., et al. (2014). Can carbohydrate mouth rinse improve performance during exercise?: a systematic review. *Nutrients* 6(1): 1–10.

8 Phillips, S.M., Van Loon, L.J. (2011). Dietary protein for athletes: from requirements to optimum adaptation. *Journal of Sports Science* 29 (Suppl): S29–S38.

9 Hartman, J.W,. Tang, J.E,. Wilkinson, S.E. (2007). Consumption of fat-free fluid milk after resistance exercise promotes greater lean mass accretion than does consumption of soy or carbohydrate in young, novice, male weightlifters. *American Journal of Clinical Nutrition* 86(2): 373–381.

10 Scientific Advisory Committee on Nutrition. (2016). *Vitamin D and Health.* www.gov.uk/government/uploads/system/uploads/attachment_data/file/537616/

SACN_Vitamin_D_and_Health_report.pdf (accessed April 2018).

11 American College of Sports Medicine: Sawka, M.N., Burke, L.M., et al. (2007). American College of Sports Medicine position stand. Exercise and fluid replacement. *Medicine and Science in Sports and Exercise* 39(2): 377–390.

12 Marshall, T.A. (2013). Preventing dental caries associated with sugar-sweetened beverages. *Journal of the American Dental Association* 144(10): 1148–1152.

13 De Oliveira, E.P., Burini, R.C., Jeukendrup, A.E. (2014). Gastrointestinal complaints during exercise: prevalence, etiology, and nutritional recommendations. *Sports Medicine* 44(Suppl. 1): S79–S85.

14 Sundgot-Borgen, J., Torstveit, M., Klungland M.S.(2004). Prevalence of eating disorders in elite athletes is higher than in the general population. *Clinical Journal of Sport Medicine* 14(1): 25–32.

15 Gabel, K.A. (2006). Special nutritional concerns for the female athlete. *Current Sports Medicine Reports* 5(4): 187–191.

16 Constantini, N.W. (2002). Medical concerns of the dancer. *Book of Abstracts, XXVII FIMS World Congress of Sports Medicine, Budapest, Hungary*, 2002: 151.

17 Mountjoy, M., Sundgot-Borgen, J., Burke, L., et al. (2014). The IOC consensus statement: beyond the female athlete triad – Relative Energy Deficiency in Sport (RED-S). *British Journal of Sports Medicine* 48(7): 491–497.

18 Gibson, P.R., Shepherd, S.J. (2010). Evidence-based dietary management of functional gastrointestinal symptoms: the FODMAP approach. *Journal of Gastroenterology Hepatology* 25(2): 252–258.

9

Oral Health, the Elite Athlete, and Performance

Ian Needleman

'Bodies of gods, teeth of yobs'
Katherine Child, Times LIVE
South Africa 14 October, 2014 [1]

9.1   Introduction

Sports medicine contains a wealth of knowledge about the health, wellbeing, and performance of elite athletes [2]. Oral health in these individuals has received much less attention until recently, although research studies were published nearly half a century ago [3]. The findings from research studies show consistently high levels of oral disease and, more recently, an impact on self-reported measures of performance. The result has been a reconsideration of oral health within elite sport, with an introduction or strengthening of strategies to promote oral health. The purpose of this chapter is to summarise the current state of knowledge about oral health in elite sport, its effect on performance, and what can be done to improve the situation. This field is developing rapidly and updates can be found on our webpages: www.ucl.ac.uk/cohp.

9.2   Oral Health in Elite Athletes

9.2.1   London 2012

Our study at the London Olympic Games in 2012 investigated oral health, its determinants, and the self-reported performance and wellbeing impacts from oral health [4]. We recruited athletes from those attending the Polyclinic (Figure 9.1), the substantial health centre providing free comprehensive healthcare to all athletes. The dental clinic was positioned on the top floor, together with optometry services (Figure 9.1). Over the duration of the games, we recruited 302 athletes and the main reason for excluding participants was if they, or their interpreter, were not able to understand the consent process. Data available for 278 athletes representing 25 sports, all five continents and with a wide distribution of developing and developed economies (Table 9.1). Their average age was 26 years. Interestingly, 46% of the athletes had not seen a dentist for at least 12 months preceding the games. Less than 5% reported current tobacco use.

9.2.1.1   London 2012 Oral Health Data
We found surprisingly high levels of the most common oral diseases in this sample of athletes (Figure 9.2). The proportions of athletes affected by these conditions were: dental caries 55%, dental erosion 45%, gingivitis 76%, and periodontitis 15%. On average, two teeth were affected by caries in each athlete (range 0–24 teeth). At least half the mouth was affected by gingivitis in 76% of the athletes and periodontitis was present in at least half the mouth in 8%. Signs of pericoronitis were present in 25 athletes (10%) of whom 10 reported pain.

Sports Dentistry: Principles and Practice, First Edition. Edited by Peter D. Fine, Chris Louca and Albert Leung.
© 2019 John Wiley & Sons Ltd. Published 2019 by John Wiley & Sons Ltd.
Companion website: www.wiley.com/go/fine/sports_dentistry

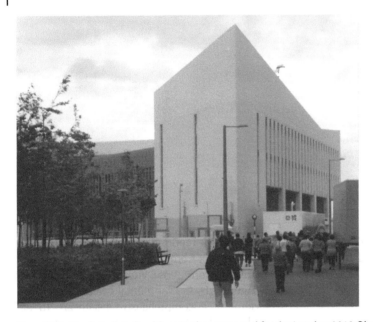

Figure 9.1 The Polyclinic (health centre) constructed for the London 2012 Olympic Games.

Table 9.1 London 2012 oral health data: participants.

	N	%
Gender	N = 278	
Male	159	57
Continent		
Africa	78	28
America	81	29
Europe	59	21
Asia	27	10
Oceania	33	12
Ethnicity	N = 250	
White	85	34
Asian	7	3
Black	79	32
Dual	41	16
Other	38	15
Sport (top 5)	N = 272	
Track and field	95	35
Boxing	38	14
Hockey	31	11
Swimming	21	8
Waterpolo	11	4

Twenty-two athletes attended due to dental or orofacial trauma (18% sample), of whom 16 were wearing mouthguards. Conducting research in the setting of a major global competition is not straightforward and requires pragmatic planning and design. As a result, the limitations to the quality of the data included the multiple examiners who carried out the oral health examinations and the severely limited opportunity for examiner training and calibration. Furthermore, because the research was carried out on a 'convenience' sample of those attending the Polyclinic, there was uncertainty as to whether the sample represented elite athletes more broadly.

9.2.2 English Professional Football 2014

The aim with our study of English professional football was to build on the research from London 2012, with the aim of achieving a representative sample [5]. We achieved this by sampling 89% or more of each of the senior squad teams that participated. The support of the eight clubs, medical teams, and attached dentists were key to ensuring good participation. The clubs included five from the Premier League, two from the

Championship, and one League One team. Overall, we collected data from 187 players, able to understand the consent process, at least 18 years of age, and in the senior squad. Examinations were conducted by the usual team dentist or one nominated by the club and took place at the teams' medical or training facilities. The majority of players were white (75%). In contrast to the London 2012 sample, only 27% reported that they had not visited a dentist within 12 months. Reported tobacco use was again low at 5%, and mostly smokeless.

9.2.2.1 Professional Football Oral Health Data

The findings from professional football again showed high levels of poor oral health with the following percentage of players affected: caries 37%, erosion 53%, gingivitis 80%, and periodontitis 5% (Figure 9.2). Experience of dental caries or restorations increased with age with DFT = 1 or more in 78% of 6–24-year-olds, but 92% of 25–34-year-old players. Pericoronitis was infrequent at 3%. However, 8% of participants had at least one PUFA finding (open pulp, ulceration, fistula, or abscess). There were clear differences in prevalence of some conditions compared

with the London 2012 Olympic data, particularly for dental caries and periodontitis. However, how much these differences are related to study methods such as the detection thresholds of the examiners cannot be determined, although they were all highly experienced dentists. In view of the mostly less than ideal examination conditions in the study, it is most likely that these values underestimated the true disease prevalence.

In the absence of a control group, we attempted to compare the data with UK population values, using the most recent Adult Dental Health Survey (ADHS) [6]. We found that footballers appeared to have more restorations and at least similar or higher levels of untreated caries. In the 16–24 years age group, the proportion of footballers with dentine caries was higher (38.3%) than the same cohort in the ADHS (30%). The proportion of footballers with one or more restorations was higher than the ADHS values: 16–24 years cohort, football 69.8%, ADHS 53%; 25–34 years cohort, football 88.3%, ADHS 75%. The mean number of teeth per participant with restorations was: 16–24 years, football 4.9, ADHS 3.4; 25–34 years, football 5.2, ADHS 5.1. Clearly, such a comparison should be interpreted with great caution due to differing research designs.

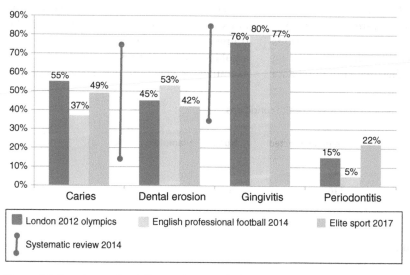

Figure 9.2 Prevalence of oral diseases in research data.

As with the London 2012 study, pragmatic research design decisions were needed. Despite the sample being representative, which was a major development from the London 2012 data, the limitations for this study were again the need to use multiple examiners (six dentists for the eight clubs) and the limited opportunity to train and calibrate them.

9.2.3 Systematic Review of Oral Health in Sport

In order to understand the research base for oral health in elite sport, we conducted a systematic review based on the focused question: What is the oral health of athletes and what is the effect of oral health on athletic training and performance? [7] We anticipated that it might be difficult to find all possibly relevant studies. As a result, we deliberately planned a sensitive search strategy, providing a high chance of finding relevant studies, but with the disadvantage of needing to screen many irrelevant ones. We searched electronically Ovid MEDLINE (1950 to October 2013), Ovid EMBASE (which has a greater emphasis on non-English language publications) (1980 to October 2013), EBSCO SPORTDiscus (up to October 2013) (for a focus on sport-related research) and OpenGrey (www.opengrey.eu) (for unpublished research). No date or language restrictions were applied. We found 9858 potentially relevant citations which were screened for relevance, leading to selection of 34 studies that contained data

for the review. Of these, most (26/34) focused on dental trauma. In the 16 studies that reported oral health data, we again found a high prevalence of oral diseases in the athletes, although with much variation between studies in methods and findings. The proportion of athletes affected by these conditions were: dental caries 15–75%, dental erosion 36–85%, periodontitis 15% (Table 9.2). The strength of the evidence was compromised by a number of factors affecting the studies, including risk of bias, lack of examiner training, and convenience sampling. As described above, these issues of research methodology reflect the difficulties of conducting sports medicine research in elite and professional settings. Systematic reviews are also useful for identifying important gaps in the research base. For this review, the most important areas lacking evidence were periodontal health and the impact of oral health on performance (see below).

9.2.4 Elite Sport Oral Health 2017 Study

Recognising the limitations in the strength of the research, we designed a new study to overcome these as far as possible [8]. The primary aims in quality improvement were the training and calibration of the examiner, combined with representative sampling. To achieve these ambitions, all clinical examinations were conducted by a single, carefully trained examiner who was calibrated against a gold standard, experienced examiner. The examiner travelled to each sport training

Table 9.2 London 2012 oral health data: oral health conditions.

Prevalence of disease	Number affected	Number in sample	%
Caries	145	263	55
Dental erosion	116	260	45
Gingivitis only	211	278	76
Periodontitis	42	278	15
New dental/orofacial trauma	22	125	17
Pericoronitis	25	253	10

centre to conduct the examinations and to collect the questionnaire data. Together with the support of the each sport organisation, we were able to achieve screening of more than 75% of each team with the exception of track and field athletics. The sports included were the following GB Olympic Teams: athletics, gymnastics, cycling, swimming, rowing, sailing, rugby 7s and hockey, as well as professional teams in football, rugby, and cycling. All athletes were senior squad athletes aged 18 years or over. To date, 352 athletes have participated in the study. The findings were highly consistent with our previous research (Figure 9.2). The proportion of athletes affected by disease was: caries 49%, erosive tooth wear 42%, gingivitis 77%, and periodontitis 22%.

9.2.5 Summary

Overall, the research base is consistent in reporting high levels of poor oral health in elite sport. It is notable that the consistency of these findings has not changed, despite more robust research designs being

employed. This suggests that the data are reliable. Figure 9.3 shows examples of severe oral health problems in elite athletes.

9.2.6 Impact on Performance

Whilst oral health is in itself an important parameter for athletes, of particular relevance to the athletes, performance directors, and funders is whether there are consequences for performance. This was a key question for us from the outset, as there are consistent data that poor oral health negatively affects wellbeing and quality of life [9]. It is clear that performance would certainly be affected by catastrophic events arising from severe acute infections (e.g. acute pericoronitis), dental and orofacial trauma, or pain from pulpitis, and these could lead to immediate losses to play (LTP). Whilst important, the data suggest that they are infrequent.

However, lower severity, chronic influences might also be important in training and performance, particularly where differences between elite performances at the top

(a)

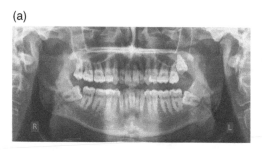

(b)

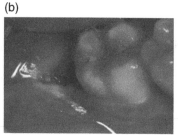

(c)

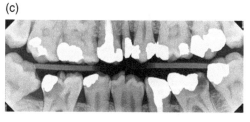

Figure 9.3 Examples of oral health problems in elite athletes. Track and field athlete with pain and swelling from acute pericoronitis. (a) Panoramic radiograph, (b) impacted, partially erupted third molar. (Images courtesy of Dr Geoff St George, Centre for Oral Health and Performance, UCL, London, UK). (c) Premier league professional footballer with severe pain showing extensive dental caries extending into dental pulp (nerve chamber). (Image courtesy of Dr Ian Hunt, Maple Dental, Manchester, UK).

end of the range differ by a small fraction of a percentage. In this concept, marginal gains/losses from more common issues such as mild to moderate pain, systemic inflammation, sleep disturbance, and emotional well-being/confidence are important elements of overall athlete preparation. Assessing these impacts as self-reported measures is widely used and valued in athlete surveillance [10]. They are recognised as having the potential to capture a broader range of impacts than clinician-assessed health outcomes or performance measures such as time loss [11].

Due to time constraints for data collection, we limited self-reported performance evaluation at London 2012 [4] to a modification of a validated global oral health quality of life tool [12]. The three questions asked athletes were:

a) To what extent have you been bothered by your oral health in the last 12 months?
b) To what extent has your oral health affected your quality of life overall in the last 12 months?
c) To what extent has your oral health affected your athletic performance or training over the last 12 months?

The responses to the questions were scored on a five-point scale:

1) Not at all
2) A little
3) Somewhat
4) A fair amount
5) A great deal.

The results were surprising (Figure 9.4). More than 40% of athletes were 'bothered' by their oral health, with 28% reporting an impact on quality of life and 18% on training and performance.

Self-reported impacts were also clear in professional football (Figure 9.4). A very high proportion of footballers were bothered by their oral health (45%) with 20% reporting an effect on their quality of life, and 7% on training and performance. For the next study, we were able to employ more detailed evaluation of self-reported impacts [8]. Of 352 athletes examined, 34% reported some impact on their training or performance due to their oral health. The psycho-social impacts are illuminating. As a result of their oral health, 35% athletes reported difficulties eating or drinking, 15% an impact on sleeping, and

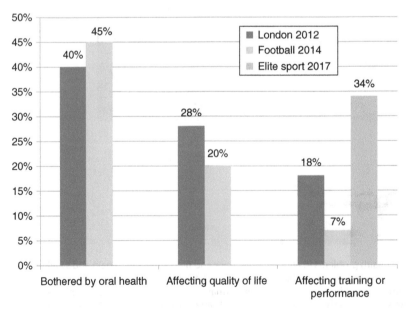

Figure 9.4 Self-reported impacts of poor oral health on athlete performance and wellbeing.

17% some difficulty in smiling, laughing, or showing teeth without embarrassment.

In addition to the above, we found three studies in the systematic review reporting data on performance impacts, although there were many issues about the interpretation of the data [7]. These issues included studies that combined responses from athletes and non-athletes together, small sample sizes, and invalidated methods. Each study, however, found negative impacts from oral health. In an evaluation at the 1992 Barcelona Olympic Games, 8% of respondents thought their oral health had affected training and 4% performance (although only 54% of the survey participants were athletes) [13]. Amongst Brazilian basketball players, 33% felt insecure about playing following sport-related orofacial trauma and 66% reported that oral problems could 'diminish their strength' [14]. A cross-sectional study of 30 footballers from Barcelona FC found an association between dental plaque index and musculoskeletal injuries. As this was cross-sectional evidence, the research could not establish causation [15].

The consistency of self-reported impacts on performance is important. If anything, it is likely that these data underestimate the impacts; some athletes may not associate impaired performance with their oral health since this has not been a priority area of awareness or routine surveillance within sports medicine. What is striking is that these athletes represent people at the pinnacle of physical and mental preparation and aspiration. It seems remarkable that such a high proportion of participants reported effects from their oral health that could undermine their performance.

9.3 Causes of Poor Oral Health in Elite Sport

9.3.1 Introduction

The determinants of oral health are complex and there is no reason to believe this is any different in elite sport. There are only few

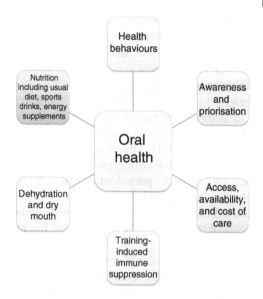

Figure 9.5 Complexity of factors determining oral health in athletes.

studies that have begun to explore this relationship and therefore, the following model is based upon what we know from the limited existing data, knowledge about health determinants more broadly in sport and an understanding of determinants of oral health outside of sport (Figure 9.5).

9.3.2 Nutrition

Nutrition is a major determinant of oral health, including daily diet, sports drinks, and supplements. Carbohydrate-containing sports drinks and gels are often used to enhance training and performance, and may be taken frequently and over long periods [16–19]. These supplements include energy drinks (normally with a CHO concentration of >10%), isotonic sports drinks (4–8% CHO) and hypotonic drinks (normally around 2% CHO or less) [20]. Dietary carbohydrate intake and caries risk is well characterised [21] and acidic intake is the main factor causing erosive tooth wear [4,22]. A relationship between dental caries and frequency of sports drink intake has been reported in children [23], but few studies have examined this relationship in the elite athlete population.

We found an association between the frequency of sports drink use and anterior tooth dental erosion, but not for caries, in Olympic athletes [4]. Frequent carbohydrate intakes have also been suggested as a cause of caries seen in elite triathletes [16].

In addition to caries, high carbohydrate intakes are recognised for their pro-inflammatory effects [24]. Therefore, it is possible that a high carbohydrate intake might also increase risk of periodontal diseases in athletes [24,25]. Whilst attention is often focused on sport supplements, they are only a part of the nutrition of athletes that might affect oral health.

Eating disorders could also have an impact on oral health in elite sport and have received very little attention. This might be expected, particularly where body weight, composition, and aesthetics are crucial factors [26–28], such as boxing, horse riding, gymnastics, and long-distance running [29]. Dentists managing athletes should look for signs and symptoms of erosive tooth wear as a result of eating disorders, as this might be the first detectable sign of these very serious conditions [30–33]. This is also discussed in Chapter 8.

9.3.3 Local and Systemic Environmental Factors

Saliva has a crucial role in maintaining oral health. The protection from saliva is likely to be compromised during sport activity that causes dehydration and local drying of the mouth, reduced salivary flow, or qualitative changes in salivary composition [34]. Athletes with prolonged periods of high air flow during training and performance might be at higher risk of impairment. An impact on oral health might then arise though reduced protection from the effects of carbohydrates on caries, acidic drinks on erosion, and dental plaque on gingivitis and periodontitis. Such protection is normally effected through non-specific and specific antimicrobial activity (also important in protection against periodontal diseases) and remineralising effects of saliva [22,35].

Exercise-induced immune suppression might also play a role in impairing protection against the microbial challenge of dental caries and periodontal disease [36].

9.3.4 Health Behaviours, Health Literacy, and Ecological Factors

The complexity of the determinants of oral health is well known [37,38]. Health behaviours, health beliefs, socioeconomic status, oral health literacy, access to preventive programmes, and prioritisation of time are all recognised as important determinants of oral health [38]. However, very little is known about these determinants in elite sport, although there are some data suggesting that awareness of risk of oral disease appears low [16]. From our data, we found that less than half of athletes sampled at London 2012 attended for regular oral health assessments [4]. Although attendance was higher in professional football at 75%, this still leaves 25% of these athletes not accessing regular care. In relation to the possible influence of ethnicity on the London 2012 data, white athletes had less caries and better periodontal health than other ethnicities. What we are unable to do is to determine whether ethnicity is the direct factor responsible for the association or whether ethnicity is instead a marker of socioeconomic status (SES), with SES being the true determinant, although this seems likely. There are clear social gradients with oral health in general populations and we would also expect this to be reflected in athlete populations to some extent [39,40].

Whilst regular attendance for dental examinations would seem desirable, it does not necessarily predict better oral health [41,42]. One of the reasons for this is that preventive care may not always be prioritised or provided, especially when remuneration is focused on treatment rather than on promoting health [41–45]. In addition, the elite athlete's special needs for prevention and health promotion may not be recognised.

The athlete's support ecosystem also deserves consideration. The oral health of athletes will be influenced, guided, or directed by this network, including fellow team members, medical, nutritional, and sports science support staff, and the related sport organisations [46,47]. Attempting to improve oral health or adherence to behaviour change within elite sport is unlikely to succeed unless the intervention is designed with an understanding of the ecology [48,49].

In summary, any consideration of elite athlete oral health should include an understanding of aspects close to the athlete, and potentially under their control, for which they can take responsibility, as well as more distant factors over which they may have less control. These factors are likely to be decisive for success and will benefit from engagement with the athlete's network of support when designing oral health interventions.

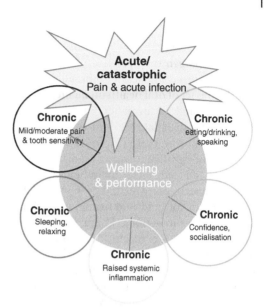

Figure 9.6 Model of mechanisms of impact of oral health on wellbeing and performance.

9.4 Causes of Performance Impacts

In a similar way to the causes of poor oral health in athletes, the causes of performance impacts are likely to be complex and again there are few data to date to provide clear direction. We propose that the causes are likely to be both a combination of severe and catastrophic, acute causes, such as acute infections and severe pain, and lower-grade, chronic causes, including less severe pain, psychosocial impacts, and potentially raised systemic inflammation(Figure 9.6).

9.4.1 Acute/Catastrophic Impacts

Acute/catastrophic impacts include causes such as significant orofacial or dental trauma, and severe pain arising from acute infections such as might be experienced with pericoronitis, acute periapical periodontitis, and irreversible pulpitis. The characteristics of these causes are that they occur infrequently, but are severe enough to prevent training or competition until resolved, and therefore will cause time loss. These are the most well-

recognised impacts of oral health on performance, even appearing in national media [50]. Alarmingly, 8% of professional footballers had at least one PUFA finding, which was either causing a catastrophic performance impact or likely to result in one in the near future without treatment [5].

9.4.2 Chronic Impacts

These impacts have received very little attention to date, possibly because they are more difficult to detect. The characteristic of chronic impacts is that in general they will not prevent training or competition (although could transition to an acute/catastrophic cause), but instead reduce an athlete's effectiveness in training or performance. They might arise from less severe pain, such as caries, reversible pulpitis, dentine hypersensitivity, from difficulties in eating and nutrition, and raised systemic inflammation resulting from oral infection. The characteristics of these impacts are that they are much more common, do not cause time loss, and may even not be directly recognised for their effect by the athlete due to their insidious onset.

9.4.3 Oral Health Performance Data

We found highly statistically significant associations between the presence of caries and athlete-reported impacts ('bothered' by oral health, impact of oral health on quality of life, or training and performance) in the London 2012 and football data [4,5]. In addition, certain self-reported oral symptoms also had a statistically significant association with athlete-reported impacts, including current pain in mouth, pain related to teeth, tooth sensitivity to hot/cold, and history of wisdom tooth swelling/infections. There were similar findings from our recent data [8]. These effects of pain or sensitivity would be consistent with a model of an impact arising from more common, chronic stimuli, since caries and sensitivity were highly prevalent. However, it is important to highlight that cross-sectional data cannot prove causation and therefore these observations remain associations.

9.4.4 Oral Health and Quality of Life

It is well recognised that oral health is a determinant of life quality (for a review see reference 8). Impacts of oral diseases on quality of life have been consistently demonstrated for caries [51], periodontal diseases [52], and pericoronitis [53]. These impacts affect peoples' lives, impairing sleeping, confidence, emotional wellbeing, and socialisation [9]. Therefore, since oral health can produce measurable psychosocial impacts, it would be surprising if training and performance were not affected in athletes with poor oral health. As we have seen earlier in the data at London 2012 and professional football, 40–45% of participants were bothered by their oral health and 20–28% reported that it was affecting their quality of life. These are highly prevalent impacts. Our latest data give further insight into these impacts (see Section 9.2.4) and the high values [8]. The high proportions of athletes who report impacts on eating and drinking,

sleeping, and difficulties in smiling is remarkable, particularly in view of how preventable these impacts should be. Caries, gingivitis, periodontitis, and erosive tooth wear could each affect these parameters, including mechanisms such as pain, sensitivity, changes to appearance, bleeding, and halitosis. Furthermore, such causes might be real or perceived [53,54]. There is therefore clear evidence of an association between oral health and negative psychosocial impacts in elite athletes. It is no coincidence that parameters are routinely assessed in elite sport (often daily) because of their importance to athlete wellbeing, performance, and risk of injury [10].

9.4.5 Systemic Inflammation

Reducing systemic inflammation and oxidative stress might improve performance and has become part of athlete health management [54,55]. Nutritional interventions are one approach that can be used [54]. Poor oral health is consistently associated with a systemic inflammatory response, particularly that arising from periodontal diseases [56]. The local inflammatory stimulus initiated by the dental plaque microbiota gives rise to a systemic response and can be measured by key inflammatory biomarkers. This is not surprising, given that the total surface area of inflamed, ulcerated epithelium can be as much as $72\,cm^2$ with severe periodontitis, similar to the surface area of the palm of the hand [57] (Figure 9.7). It is notable that within our clinical studies we have found the prevalence of periodontitis to be up to 20% and in view of the screening tool used, this is likely to underestimate true prevalence values. Furthermore, other causes of raised systemic inflammation from oral conditions could include endodontic infections and pericoronitis, both of which were present in elite athlete populations. Therefore, the findings of poor oral health in the research studies are likely to induce increased systemic inflammation in

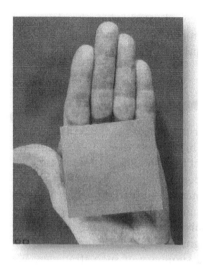

Figure 9.7 Illustration of estimated total surface area of ulcer within combined periodontal pockets in a person with generalised moderate to severe chronic periodontitis. The square on the palm represents the combined size of ulcerated epithelium [56]. (Reproduced with permission from the American Academy of Periodontology.)

affected athletes. Although the increased inflammatory burden arising from oral infection has not been measured in athletes, these conditions must be treated (and preferably prevented) as they can otherwise lead to irreversible effects on health and wellbeing.

9.4.6 Summary

In summary, poor oral health can affect performance catastrophically though severe pain and acute infections arising from disease conditions and these are likely to be infrequent occurrences. More frequent will be the prevalent, more subtle impacts that arise from mild to moderate pain and sensitivity, from the common psycho-social impacts of poor oral health, and potentially from increased systemic inflammation. Because of the lack of awareness of oral health in sport, these may be less evident to athletes themselves and under-reported. In elite sport where 'marginal

gains' are critical, oral health might therefore be one of a number of important determinants of performance.

9.5 Interventions for Athlete Oral Health

We have seen so far that there are high levels of caries, erosive tooth wear, and periodontal diseases in athletes. This section will consider the interventions required to promote oral health, prevent disease, and mitigate risk in the elite sport population.

9.5.1 Periodic Dental Health Assessments (PDHA) by Dental Professionals

There is a clear need to provide regular examinations/screening of athletes in view of the data showing the high levels of dental disease [20]. These assessments are required to both identify and provide any required treatment. The research in professional football [5] led to a call to action to implement regular examinations, as the evidence suggested a greater priority than existed for the regular musculoskeletal screening that is currently provided [58]. These examinations should be twice per year, preferably during a pre-season period (if relevant to the sport) and at one other time base on the risk profile of athletes. There is some evidence that Premier League clubs in England are adopting such a strategy [59]. The priority for these PDHAs is to identify disease and provide treatment, but they will also provide an opportunity to reinforce preventive oral health behaviours. A comprehensive oral health assessment by a dentist will be required, including dental caries, erosive tooth wear, and periodontal diseases (as a minimum a basic periodontal examination [60]), and, in view of the high caries rate, it is likely that many athletes will require radiographs as a supplement to the clinical examination for caries. Furthermore, assessment of possible pericoronitis will be important in view of the athlete age group and the potential for significant impact on performance. The clinician should also be sensitive to the potential of eating disorders, especially bulimia, to be the first detectable sign of this potentially life-threatening condition. Certain sports may also increase the risk of gastroesophageal reflux disease (GORD) [61], although the evidence for erosive tooth wear in athletes related to GORD is unclear [62,63]. Assessment, preferably during a pre-season window will then allow for necessary treatment to be provided, minimising impact on key season goals. Screening will be covered further in Chapter 10.

9.5.2 Oral Health Promotion in Athletes

Overall, the strategy most likely to be successful will be to embed oral health promotion within overall athlete care and wellbeing [48]. Many of the strategies that promote oral health are also shared across other aspects of athlete care, but may need further refinement for maximum impact on oral health. Nutrition is a major element in athlete preparation and wellbeing. Emphasising good nutrition for health, outside of performance and training directly, will include the avoidance of sugars other than the carbohydrates recommended for optimum sport performance. Similarly, avoidance of potentially acidic intakes outside of performance/training needs will be beneficial, including acidic sports beverages, fruit juices, and carbonated drinks, whether sugar-containing or not. Culturally, dental assessments should be included as part of the standard periodic health assessments that athletes undertake, especially pre-season. Scheduling the examinations by the support team will help to ensure these take place at a convenient time and preferably in a convenient location, both of which will promote uptake. Buy-in by the support team (medical, nutritional, physiotherapy, performance director, etc.) will also

favour a coordinated strategy when oral health is embedded and therefore not separate and optional.

9.5.3 Disease Prevention and Risk Mitigation

Prevention of dental diseases is well described [71]. The high levels of disease in athletes suggest that they should be viewed as at high risk until demonstrated otherwise from successive clinical examinations [20]. However, since training and performance may vary considerably during any period, risk stratification might be highly dynamic. Table 9.3 provides a summary of such strategies. We have adapted current guidance for caries, erosive tooth wear, periodontal diseases, and others to consider particular sport characteristics and the full toolkit can be downloaded at www.ucl.ac.uk/COHP. Inspired by the Team Sky concept 'the bed in a bag' [64], we have also designed a 'gob in a bag' kit to provide athletes with everything needed for their oral care (Figure 9.8). Our rationale was that adherence was more likely if we provided all that was needed, rather than expecting the athlete or team to find the items, and feedback has been very positive. Clearly, guidance does change with time and there should be a plan in place for when to check for updates. Also of relevance is that guidance for oral health promotion varies internationally and, in addition, availability of products and their specification varies in different countries.

In addition to classic disease prevention, risk mitigation should also be considered an important strategy for athlete oral health. For instance, carbohydrate intakes are essential in many sports to support training and achieve optimal performance [18]. Furthermore, in endurance sports, these supplements, which might also be acidic, risking erosive tooth wear, may be required repeatedly over long periods of activity [19]. Consequently, it will be important to understand these factors and devise strategies to attempt to reduce their impact on oral

Table 9.3 Examples of oral health prevention actions. This is not a comprehensive toolkit but illustrates some of the possible actions. Note, there is much overlap and where one action may help other conditions, this is not duplicated. (Based on *Delivering Better Oral Health* 3rd Edition [71].

	Action
General	*Embed oral health promotion within athlete care.* Include regular oral health assessments, education and behaviour change. Consider the ecological network of the athlete including local sport medicine, nutrition and performance support team as well as higher level policy makers and funders.
Dental caries	*Reduce sugar amount and frequency where feasible,* both within and outside of sport activity. For example water, milk of hypotonic sports drinks for hydration rather than higher sugar beverages. Use toothpaste with at least 1400 ppm fluoride and preferably 5000 ppm.
Erosive tooth-wear	*Reduce frequency of acidic dietary intakes including sports drinks where feasible.* Avoid prolonged retention in the mouth, rinse with after afterwards or use straw to drink if possible.
Periodontal diseases	*Brush twice per day for at least two minutes, clean between the teeth once per day before brushing and seek instruction from a dental care professional.* Avoid tobacco use.

(a)

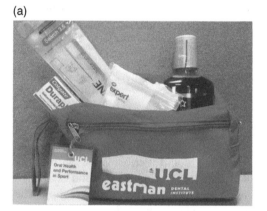

(b)

Figure 9.8 (a) 'Gob in a bag' kit. Including key items for oral health care for athletes with recommended minimum athlete 'drills'. (b) Athlete drills.

health if possible (for summary see Table 9.3). There are very few studies yet published to investigate the benefits of risk mitigation approaches in athletes. This means that such strategies can be only considered 'good practice points' for the present time and should be evaluated in research. However, there is evidence that isotonic sports drinks may differ in their erosive potential [65–67] and careful selection of products may be helpful. To complicate this issue further, in some studies, products with lower erosive potential were considered less palatable, which might compromise adherence [66].

9.5.4 Health Behaviour Change in Sport

Preventing oral diseases frequently requires health behaviour change, such as encouraging attendance for oral health examinations, the use of high-fluoride toothpastes, practising more effective oral hygiene, or reducing intake of sugars not required for sport. It would be simplistic to consider the athlete in isolation when planning these behaviour change interventions, but as introduced earlier, the athlete is at the centre of a network that might potentially either enhance or limit the potential for behaviour change. Therefore, consideration of these factors can help to design interventions with a greater chance of sustained change [68]. A further useful guide has been produced by the International Olympic Committee that emphasises the importance of integrating the behaviour change with the network and systems involving the athlete [69]. For instance, accessibility to dental professionals might limit the uptake of oral health screening, despite recommended policy. Identifying the barriers and implementing a policy such as setting up oral health screening at the same time as other health screening procedures would be helpful. Where not possible, scheduling oral health assessments within an appropriate phase of the training/performance cycle with a dental professional recognised as part of and reporting to the team,

would integrate, facilitate, and likely promote uptake. Interestingly, where comprehensive periodic screening of athletes is conducted, oral health may not be considered [70].

Another example is the use of repeated carbohydrate energy supplements during endurance sport. Where feasible, for example on long cycle training sessions or looped or track-side events, providing water alone for hydration following carbohydrate intake might help to reduce the duration of cariogenic activity within the mouth. Providing the instruction is one element, providing the kit is another and developing buy-in and agreeing joint strategies with the athletes, nutritionists, and other team support staff will also help to encourage implementation.

9.6 Centre for Oral Health and Performance

In recognition of the importance of oral health in sport, we established the Centre for Oral Health and Performance within the UCL (University College London) Eastman Dental Institute (www.ucl.ac.uk/cohp). The Centre provides a focus for research, information and awareness, training and education, and clinical care for oral health in sport. We also recognise that there are many individuals with an interest in this topic across the fields of oral health, sport and exercise medicine, and nutrition, and our network provides a means to connect people.

9.7 Summary

Research shows that the oral health of elite athletes is poor, with high levels of preventable conditions. Typically, a fifth of athletes also report a negative impact of their oral health on training and performance and this is likely to underestimate the real effect. Many of these athletes have impacts on sleeping, eating, smiling, and wellbeing.

Promoting and maintaining oral health should be considered a priority within elite sport in view of the wellbeing and performance impacts and the simple, low-cost strategies that are available with proven evidence of effectiveness. Embedding oral health within overall athlete health will be key to achieving sustained improvements.

Acknowledgements

The author would like to thank the many athletes, teams, organisations, sport and exercise medicine clinicians and scientists, and dentists who participated in or facilitated the research.

References

1 Child, K. (2014). Bodies of gods, teeth of yobs. www.timeslive.co.za/thetimes/2014/10/14/Bodies-of-gods-teeth-of-yobs1 (accessed June 2018).

2 Brukner, P. Khan, K. (2017). *Clinical Sports Medicine*. McGraw Hill Education, Australia: 1056.

3 Forrest, J.O. (1969). Dental condition of Olympic Games contestants - a pilot study. *Dental Practitioner and Dental Record* 20: 95–101.

4 Needleman, I., Ashley, P., Petrie, A., et al. (2013). Oral health and impact on performance of athletes participating in the London 2012 Olympic Games: a cross-sectional study. *British Journal of Sports Medicine* 47: 1054–1058.

5 Needleman, I., Ashley, P., Meehan, L., et al. (2016). Poor oral health including active caries in 187 UK professional male football players: clinical dental examination performed by dentists. *British Journal of Sports Medicine* 50: 41–44.

6 White, D., Pitts, N., Steele, J., Sadler, K., Chadwick, B. (2011). Disease and related disorders: a report from the Adult Dental Health Survey 2009. In: *Adult Dental Health Survey 2009: Summary report and thematic series* (ed. O'Sullivan, I.). Health and Social Care Information Centre: 1–55.

7 Ashley, P., Di Iorio, A., Cole, E., Tanday, A., Needleman, I. (2015). Oral health of elite athletes and association with performance: a systematic review. *British Journal of Sports Medicine* 49: 14–19.

8 Gallagher, J., Ashley, P., Petrie, A., Needleman, I. (in press). Oral health and impact on performance in elite and professional sport. Community Dentistry & Oral Epidemiology.

9 Locker, D. (1988). Measuring oral health: a conceptual framework. *Community Dental Health* 5: 5–13.

10 Gallagher, J., Needleman, I., Ashley, P., Sanchez, R.G., Lumsden, R. (2016). Self-reported outcome measures of the impact of injury and illness on athlete performance: a systematic review. *Sports Medicine*: 1–14. Sports Medcine ePub10.1007/s40279-016-0651-5

11 Saw, A.E., Main, L.C., Gastin, P B. (2016). Monitoring the athlete training response: subjective self-reported measures trump commonly used objective measures: a systematic review. *British Journal of Sports Medicine* 50: 281–291.

12 Locker, D., Quinonez, C. (2011). To what extent do oral disorders compromise the quality of life? *Community Dentistry and Oral Epidemiology* 39: 3–11.

13 Soler, B.D., Batchelor, P.A., Sheiham, A. (1994). The prevalence of oral health problems in participants of the 1992 Olympic Games in Barcelona. *International Dental Journal* 44: 44–48.

14 Frontera, R.R., Zanin, L., Ambrosano, G.M., Florio, F.M. (2011). Orofacial trauma in Brazilian basketball players and level of information concerning trauma and mouthguards. *Dental Traumatology* 27: 208–216.

15 Gay-Escoda, C., Vieira-Duarte-Pereira, D.M., Ardevol, J., et al. (2011). Study of the effect of oral health on physical condition of professional soccer players of the Football Club Barcelona. *Medicina Oral, Patologia Oral Y Cirugia Bucal* 16: e436–e439.

16 Bryant, S., McLaughlin, K., Morgaine, K., Drummond, B. (2011). Elite athletes and oral health. *International Journal of Sports Medicine* 32: 720–724.

17 Lun, V., Erdman, K.A., Fung, T.S., Reimer, R.A. (2012). Dietary supplementation practices in Canadian high-performance athletes. *International Journal of Sport Nutrition and Exercise Metabolism* 22: 31–37.

18 Burke, L.M., Hawley, J.A., Wong, S.H.S., Jeukendrup, A.E. (2011). Carbohydrates for training and competition. *Journal of Sports Sciences* 29(Suppl. 1): S17–S27.

19 Jeukendrup, A.E. (2011). Nutrition for endurance sports: marathon, triathlon, and road cycling. *Journal of Sports Sciences* 29(Suppl. 1): S91–S99.

20 Needleman, I., Ashley, P., Fine, P., et al. (2014). Consensus statement: oral health and elite sport performance. *British Dental Journal* 217: 587–590.

21 Moynihan, P.J., Kelly, S.A. (2014). Effect on caries of restricting sugars intake: systematic review to inform WHO guidelines. *Journal of Dental Research* 93: 8–18.

22 Lussi, A., Jaeggi, T., Zero, D. (2004). The role of diet in the aetiology of dental erosion. *Caries Research* 38(Suppl 1): 34–44.

23 Kawashita, Y., Fukuda, H., Kawasaki, K., et al. (2011). Pediatrician-recommended use of sports drinks and dental caries in 3-year-old children. *Community Dental Health* 28: 29–33.

24 Chapple, I.L.C. (2009). Potential mechanisms underpinning the nutritional modulation of periodontal inflammation. *Journal of the American Dental Association* 140: 178–184.

25 Baumgartner, S., Imfeld, T., Schicht, O., et al. (2009). The impact of the Stone Age diet on gingival conditions in the absence of oral hygiene. *Journal of Periodontology* 80: 759–768.

26 Ackland, T.R., Lohman, T.G., Sundgot-Borgen, J., et al. (2012). Current status of body composition assessment in sport: review and position statement on behalf of the Ad Hoc Research Working Group on Body Composition Health and Performance, under the auspices of the I.O.C. Medical Commission. *Sports Medicine* 42: 227–249.

27 Sundgot-Borgen, J., Garthe, I. (2011). Elite athletes in aesthetic and Olympic weight-class sports and the challenge of body weight and body compositions. *Journal of Sports Sciences*, 29(Suppl. 1): S101–S114.

28 Sundgot-Borgen, J., Meyer, N.L., Lohman, T.G., et al. (2013). How to minimise the health risks to athletes who compete in weight-sensitive sports review and position statement on behalf of the Ad Hoc Research Working Group on Body Composition, Health and Performance, under the auspices of the IOC Medical Commission. *British Journal of Sports Medicine* 47: 1012–1022.

29 Sundgot-Borgen, J., Torstveit, M.K. (2004). Prevalence of eating disorders in elite athletes is higher than in the general population. *Clinical Journal of Sport Medicine* 14: 25–32.

30 Walsh, J.M.E., Wheat, M.E., Freund, K. (2000). Detection, evaluation, and treatment of eating disorders. *Journal of General Internal Medicine* 15: 577–590.

31 Hermont, A.P., Pordeus, I.A., Paiva, S.M., Abreu, M.H.N.G.Ú., Auad, S.M.Í. (2013). Eating disorder risk behavior and dental implications among adolescents.

International Journal of Eating Disorders 46: 677–683.

32 Hermont, A.P., Oliveira, P.A.D., Martins, C.C., et al. (2014). Tooth erosion and eating disorders: a systematic review and meta-analysis. *PLoS One* 9, e111123.

33 Fairbrother, T. (2016). My eating disorder enarly ended my marathon dreams – but now I'm back up and running. The Running Blog. *The Guardian Newspaper*. www.theguardian.com/lifeandstyle/the-running-blog/2016/jan/08/my-eating-disorder-nearly-ended-my-marathon-dreams-but-now-im-back-up-and-running (accessed April 2018).

34 Mulic, A., Tveit, A.B., Songe, D., Sivertsen, H., Skaare, A. (2012). Dental erosive wear and salivary flow rate in physically active young adults. *BMC Oral Health* 12: 8.

35 Allaker, R.P., Ian Douglas, C.W. (2015). Non-conventional therapeutics for oral infections. *Virulence* 6: 196–207.

36 Gleeson, M. (2007). Immune function in sport and exercise. *Journal of Applied Physiology* 103: 693–699.

37 Sheiham, A., Watt, R.G. (2000). The common risk factor approach: a rational basis for promoting oral health. *Community Dentistry and Oral Epidemiology* 28: 399–406.

38 Watt, R.G. (2002). Emerging theories into the social determinants of health: implications for oral health promotion. *Community Dentistry and Oral Epidemiology* 30: 241–247.

39 Sabbah, W., Tsakos, G., Chandola, T., Sheiham, A., Watt, R.G. (2007). Social gradients in oral and general health. *Journal of Dental Research* 86: 992–996.

40 Watt, R.G., Listl, S., Peres, M., Heilmann, A. (2015). Social inequalities in oral health: from evidence to action. media.news.health.ufl.edu/misc/cod-oralhealth/docs/posts.../SocialInequalities.pdf (accessed April 2018).

41 Hill, K.B., Chadwick, B., Freeman, R., O'Sullivan, I., Murray, J.J. (2013). Adult Dental Health Survey 2009: relationships between dental attendance patterns, oral health behaviour and the current barriers to dental care. *British Dental Journal* 214: 25–32.

42 Riley, P., Worthington, H.V., Clarkson, J.E., Beirne, P.V. (2013). Recall intervals for oral health in primary care patients. [Update *of Cochrane Database of Systematic Reviews 2007*;(4):CD004346; PMID: 17943814]. *Cochrane Database of Systematic Reviews* 12: CD004346.

43 Richards, W. (2008) Prevention in practice. *British Dental Journal* 205: 111.

44 Sbaraini, A. (2012) What factors influence the provision of preventive care by general dental practitioners? *British Dental Journal* 212: E18.

45 Yokoyama, Y., Kakudate, N., Sumida, F., et al. (2013). Dentists practice patterns regarding caries prevention: results from a dental practice-based research network. *British Medical Journal Open* 3(9): e003227.

46 Steffen, K., Soligard, T., Engebretsen, L. (2012). Health protection of the Olympic athlete. *British Journal of Sports Medicine* 46: 466–470.

47 Geidne, S., Quennerstedt, M., Eriksson, C. (2013). The youth sports club as a health-promoting setting: An integrative review of research. *Scandinavian Journal of Public Health* 41: 269–283.

48 Dijkstra, H.P., Pollock, N., Chakraverty, R., Alonso, J.M. (2014). Managing the health of the elite athlete: a new integrated performance health management and coaching model. *British Journal of Sports Medicine* 48: 523–531.

49 Verhagen, E., Voogt, N., Bruinsma, A., Finch, C.F. (2014). A knowledge transfer scheme to bridge the gap between science and practice: an integration of existing research frameworks into a tool for practice. *British Journal of Sports Medicine* 48: 698–701.

50 Daily Mirror. (2014). Mo Farah lifts lid on terrifying medical emergency which led to Commonwealth games withdrawal. www.mirror.co.uk/sport/other-sports/athletics/

mo-farah-lifts-lid-terrifying-4038223 (accessed April 2018).

51 Foster Page, L.A., Thomson, W.M. (2012). Caries prevalence, severity, and 3-year increment, and their impact upon New Zealand adolescents' oral-health-related quality of life. *Journal of Public Health Dentistry* 72: 287–294.

52 Needleman, I., McGrath, C., Floyd, P., Biddle, A. (2004). Impact of oral health on the life quality of periodontal patients. *Journal of Clinical Periodontology* 31: 454–457.

53 McNutt, M., Partrick, M., Shugars, D.A., Phillips, C., White, R.P., Jr. (2008). Impact of symptomatic pericoronitis on health-related quality of life. *Journal of Oral and Maxillofacial Surgery* 66: 2482–2487.

54 Ferreira, L.F., Reid, M.B. (2008). Muscle-derived ROS and thiol regulation in muscle fatigue. *Journal of Applied Physiology* 104: 853–860.

55 Mickleborough, T.D. (2013). Omega-3 polyunsaturated fatty acids in physical performance optimization. *International Journal of Sport Nutrition and Exercise Metabolism* 23: 83–96.

56 Graziani, F., Cei, S., Orlandi, M., et al. (2015). Acute-phase response following full-mouth versus quadrant non-surgical periodontal treatment: a randomized clinical trial. *Journal of Clinical Periodontology* 42: 843–852.

57 Page, R.C. (1998). The pathobiology of periodontal diseases may affect systemic diseases: inversion of a paradigm. *Annals of Periodontology* 3, 108–120.

58 Needleman, I., Ashley, P., Weiler, R., McNally, S. (2016). Oral health screening should be routine in professional football: a call to action for sports and exercise medicine (SEM) clinicians. *British Journal of Sports Medicine* 50: 1295–1296.

59 The Sun (2016) Kick in the teeth. Manchester United boss Jose Mourinho makes use of his unique training drill ahead of new season. www.thesun.co.uk/

news/1526293/manchester-united-boss-jose-mourinho-launches-unique-training-drill-ahead-of-new-season/ (accessed April 2018).

60 British Society of Periodontology. (2016). *Basic Periodontal Examination.* www.bsperio.org.uk (accessed April 2018).

61 Parmelee-Peters, K., Moeller, J.L. (2004). Gastroesophageal reflux in athletes. *Current Sports Medicine Reports* 3: 107–111.

62 Baghele, O.N., Majumdar, I.A., Thorat, M.S., et al. (2013). Prevalence of dental erosion among young competitive swimmers: a pilot study. *Compendium of Continuing Education in Dentistry* 34: e20–e24.

63 Zebrauskas, A., Birskute, R., Maciulskiene, V. (2014). Prevalence of dental erosion among the young regular swimmers in Kaunas, Lithuania. *Journal of Oral and Maxillofacial Research* 5: e6.

64 Guardian Online (2010) Team Sky Tour de France. www.theguardian.com/sport/2010/jul/18/team-sky-tour-de-france (accessed April 2018).

65 Meurman, J.H., Harkonen, M., Naveri, H., et al. (1990). Experimental sports drinks with minimal dental erosion effect. *European Journal of Oral Sciences* 98: 120–128.

66 Cochrane, N.J., Yuan, Y., Walker, G.D., et al. (2012). Erosive potential of sports beverages. *Australian Dental Journal* 57: 359–364.

67 Ostrowska, A., Szymanski, W., Kolodziejczyk, L., Boltacz-Rzepkowska, E. (2016). Evaluation of the erosive potential of selected isotonic drinks: in vitro studies. *Advances in Clinical and Experimental Medicine* 25: 1313–1319.

68 Michie, S., van Stralen, M., West, R. (2011). The behaviour change wheel: A new method for characterising and designing behaviour change interventions. *Implementation Science* 6: 42.

69 Matheson, G.O., Klogl, M., Engebretsen, L., et al. (2013). Prevention and management of non-communicable disease: the IOC consensus statement, Lausanne 2013. *British Journal of Sports Medicine* 47: 1003–1011.

70 Bakken, A., Targett, S., Bere, T., et al. (2016). Health conditions detected in a comprehensive periodic health evaluation of 558 professional football players. *British Journal of Sports Medicine* 50: 1142–1150.

71 Public Health England. (2014). Delivering better oral health: an evidence-based toolkit for prevention, 3rd edition. www.gov.uk/government/uploads/system/uploads/attachment_data/file/367563/DBOHv32014OCTMainDocument_3.pdf (accessed April 2018).

10

Screening for Dental Disease Amongst Elite Athletes
Lyndon Meehan

10.1 Dental Care of the Sportsperson

Despite their superior fitness and conditioning, elite athletes are not immune from dental diseases. With training and participation in some sports there may be an increased susceptibility to certain types of dental conditions, notably dental caries, periodontal disease, and tooth surface loss. It is therefore imperative that athletes and sports clubs undertake and instigate regular pre-season dental screening and oral health assessments. This will inform sports medics and coaching staff on the dental status of their players or athletes. At present this author feels this is a neglected area of sports medicine that requires further highlighting.

As dental health professionals we sometimes can be solely focused on teeth, yet appreciation must be shown to the fact that athletes need to be optimally hydrated for maximum performance. In certain sports, such as rugby, basketball, and soccer, due to the changeable nature of exertion demands in the game, an athlete's metabolic needs will vary during game time. They will frequently inter-change between running, walking, and sprinting many times over the course of a game.

The best possible nutrition is essential for powering young athletes involved in sport, but also to achieve maximum growth and development. Optimal children's teeth development is determined by nutritional demands and their dietary nutritional adequacy plays a crucial role in this development [1].

However, with prolonged and sustained periods of exercise, large volumes of fluid are lost. This results in decreased blood glucose levels and depleted muscle glycogen stores, leading to dehydration, a decreased performance, and increased fatigue. Usually carbohydrates or electrolyte drinks and energy bars are consumed to maintain blood glucose levels, as high rates of carbohydrate oxidation provide an increased endurance capacity. Therefore, as a consequence of these nutritional demands, an athlete's dentition can be placed under a constant, potentially detrimental state. If left unmonitored this could have disastrous irreversible dental effects, which can impact on the athlete's ability to train, compete, and perform optimally. Athletes at every level train hard in preparation to be 'competition ready'. Therefore, the team dentist has an increasingly important role to play in the sports medicine wheel for complete athlete preparation and readiness. By undertaking pre-season or pre-competition screens, dental conditions that may influence an athlete's participation and concentration can be identified and evaluated well in advance.

This chapter shall allude to the current published evidence for poor dental health in

Sports Dentistry: Principles and Practice, First Edition. Edited by Peter D. Fine, Chris Louca and Albert Leung.
© 2019 John Wiley & Sons Ltd. Published 2019 by John Wiley & Sons Ltd.
Companion website: www.wiley.com/go/fine/sports_dentistry

sport. Practical considerations and hurdles in establishing, and how to establish a dental health screening program within modern sport shall be outlined through this author's own experience using supporting literature.

10.2 Exercise Effects on the Oral Cavity

Oral dehydration with a decreased salivary flow is a result of increased competition and energy expenditure during sport. Many of the high-carbohydrate sports drinks consumed are acidic in nature, being of a relatively low pH. Over a time period, frequent ingestion of food and drinks of a lower pH means the oral cavity remains at a lower pH for longer. Chander and Rees [2] outline that the crucial destructive pH range for enamel dissolution ranges from 4.5–5.5. A drop in the intra-oral pH value is demonstrated and represented in Figure 10.1 – the Stephan curve.

If beverages rich in carbohydrate are consumed regularly over multiple daily training sessions, to maintain adequate nutritional and hydration intake, this is the perfect breeding ground for a multitude of dental pathologies, which maintain a lower intra-oral pH for longer. Therefore to maintain a neutral pH, and thereby prevent demineralization of tooth tissue, the potential challenge faced by the dental professional is huge. Russell's study [3] on the diet of professional youth soccer players, found their total carbo-hydrate intake was inadequate, representing around 56%. Russell suggested soccer players should ideally maintain a total dietary intake comprising 60–70% carbohydrate.

This highlights the challenge dental professionals face when dealing with athletes of all abilities and all age groups. Mixed messages given to the athlete from differing sporting professions, by different personnel involved in their wellbeing, can give conflicting advice, which often pulls in differing directions. This can be confusing at best and potentially disastrous at worst.

10.3 Associated Dental Diseases

The hours of investment and struggle to achieve a heightened level of fitness and readiness to compete should not be compromised by preventable oral health problems presenting before or during competition. Therefore, regular dental screening, effective dietary advice and oral health education and prevention will have a vital role to play in the long-term health and wellbeing of athletes.

Many athletes embark upon sport at a very young age, having lengthy careers, be it professionally, semi-professionally, or purely for recreation. In the young athlete, multiple games or events and training sessions can be attended per week. This may result in a tendency to 'snack' during journeys and training, relying on sugary items to replace spent energy. If the appropriate advice and

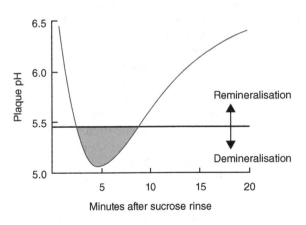

Figure 10.1 The Stephan curve (from www.wrigleysoralhealthcare.co.uk).

prevention is not outlined in the infancy of a sporting career regarding diet and nutrition in order to instil good habits, multiple irreversible dental problems may be seen.

Common dental diseases can manifest as tooth surface loss, dental caries, and periodontal disease, which may severely compromise the longevity and restorative status of a patient's dentition in later life. The aim should be to minimise the need for complex restorative intervention at a young age through good oral health measures education and advice. These specific diseases in relation to the sports person shall now be outlined.

10.4   Tooth Surface Loss

This is the gradual loss of tooth surface due to a repetitious physical contact or due to chemical dissolution. It can be caused by abrasion, abfraction, attrition, and erosion. However, it is commonly multi-factorial in nature.

10.4.1   Abfraction

This is the pathological loss of tooth structure due to biomechanical forces such as flexure, compression, or tension. Cervical V-shaped notches are commonly seen in teeth.

10.4.2   Attrition

This is a loss of tooth tissue by means of friction from tooth contacts or from restorations during biting and chewing. Flattened incisal edges and occlusal surfaces are classically seen.

10.4.3   Abrasion

This is the loss of tooth tissue by means of friction, caused by the contact of teeth with objects other than teeth. The most common cause is over-zealous brushing on exposed dentine with highly abrasive toothpastes [2,4].

10.4.4   Erosion

This is attributed to the chemical dissolution of a tooth's hard tissue not involving bacteria degradation. Tooth surfaces tend to demonstrate a shiny/glassy/stain-free appearance with rounded edges. A classic anatomical change in the tooth is the translucent incisal edge and first molar occlusal pitting. Amalgam restorations may stand proud from the tooth structure, due to the dissimilar rates of erosion between the tooth and the restorative material. Erosive sources can be intrinsic or extrinsic in nature, which shall be outlined.

Sirimaharaj et al. [5] allude to studies that have shown erosion rates amongst adults and children, to be estimated at between 2–18% of the population, and are on the increase. Common symptoms and clinical findings from tooth surface loss are summarized further in Table 10.1 below.

Images showing characteristics of tooth surface loss are presented in Figures 10.2 and 10.3.

It is difficult to be precise about the exact cause of tooth surface loss, as commonly it is multi-factorial and a combination of all of the above exists. This is due to the initial

Table 10.1 Common signs and symptoms of tooth surface loss.

Dentine hypersensitivity, characterized by short sharp pain from exposed dentine in response to thermal changes	Shortened tooth height Altered natural tooth anatomical structure
Sharp edges on teeth and tooth translucency	Unaesthetic dentition appearance Decreased facial height
Oral soft tissue trauma and ulceration	Altered dietary regime / abrasive elements
Pulpitis	Change and adaptation of masticatory function
Habitual bruxism /nail chewing	Iatrogenic damage from opposing porcelain crowns

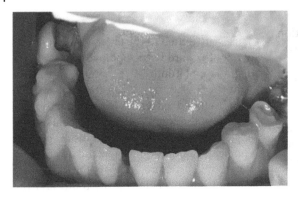
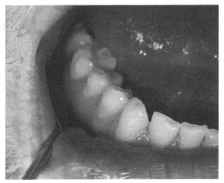

Figure 10.2 Occlusal pitting and altered tooth anatomy with sharp edges and buccal abrasion lesions.

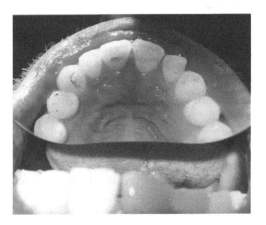

Figure 10.3 Palatal view of tooth surface loss with incisal edge pitting anteriorly.

softening and morphological change of the tooth's surface by erosion from an acidic challenge. This therefore makes a tooth more susceptible to wear and loss of structure from abrasion and attrition.

10.5 Tooth Structure

The outer surface of a tooth is a highly protective mineralized enamel layer, which covers the inner dentine structure. A thick dentine layer forms the bulk of a tooth's mineralised tissues. The tooth's root surface is covered by cementum, which aids attachment of teeth to a bony socket. At the center of a tooth is the unmineralised dental pulp, and this contains the neural and vascular network to connect the tooth with the surrounding tissues, the periodontal ligament, and the bony socket. Dentine is less mineralised than enamel and therefore more susceptible to acid erosion once the harder outer enamel layer of the tooth has been breached. Dissolution rates of dentine are reported to be three times greater than that of enamel at pH 5 [4].

10.6 The Acidic Challenge

10.6.1 Extrinsic Sources

Extrinsic sources of acidic challenges may include any athlete's dietary habits, which can include drink swishing, lifestyle factors, and the nature of their sport's nutritional demands. Sirimaharaj et al. [5] found that running, and ball and field sports had the greatest frequency of consumption of fruit juices, soft drinks, and sports drinks between meals due to their high energy expenditure and high carbohydrate need. Athletes consuming fruit juices more than twice daily were more likely to report erosion than those not consuming fruit juice.

Many fruits contain several organic acids in combination, the most prevalent being citric, malic, and oxalic acids. Citric acid is this most destructive, with the highest potential for dental erosion. High citric acid contents are found in oranges, lemons, and grapefruits [4].

Enamel dissolution from sports drinks and energy drinks is shown to be 3–11 times greater than that from cola drinks [6]. Rees found that herbal teas had an erosive effect on enamel that is five times that of traditional teas [4].

There are several published reports that indicate sportspersons who spend lengthy training times in a swimming pool, such as swimmers, water polo players, and divers, have a heightened risk for dental erosion [7–10]. Gas chlorination or sodium hypochlorite are the two main swimming pool water disinfection techniques. Chlorine compounds dissolve in water, changing the pH level. Dawes et al. [8] reported a complete loss of the enamel of anterior teeth in a person who swam daily for two weeks in an improperly chlorinated swimming pool. Dental erosion rates amongst swimmers was reported by Buczkowska-Radlinska et al. [7] and Zebrauskas et al. [10] as being between 26% and 90% of a swim team. Dental erosion has been demonstrated mainly in studies undertaken in gas-chlorinated swimming pools, rather than sodium hypochlorite-disinfected pools, where only 0.14% of pools had a pH level lower than 5.5, which would cause dental demineralisation [7,8,10,11].

D'Ercole et al. [9] carried out a study of young swimmers and reported swimming pool water with a daily pH of 7.2, which met the required pH value range from 7.20 to 9.0 and thereby had little to no effect in the development of erosion. Milosevic et al. [12] reported tooth surface loss into dentine from sports drinks use in the majority of cyclists and swimmers they studied. Cyclists, however, had a greater level of maxillary arch palatal tooth surface loss. This was attributed to an increased consumption need and a differing ingestion pattern of lower pH sports drinks.

10.6.2 Intrinsic Sources

In modern day sport, due to the potential huge media attention and copying of idols, there are sometimes pressures of striving for body perfection or in certain sports, weight restrictions may apply. Intrinsic acidic sources may be seen as intentional gastric regurgitation or an induction of vomiting as a result of prolonged strenuous exercise. This gives re-entry of gastric acids into the oral cavity, which can be highly destructive on enamel in a dehydrated mouth. The need for questioning on conditions such as alcoholism, anorexia, bulimia, and anorexia athletica should considered when dentally screening, treating, and assessing sportspersons. They all will have a drastic effect on young athletes in that their body mass growth and development will be affected, as well as performance. Ranalli [13] and Studen- Pavlovich et al. [1] detailed these conditions and outlined that the 'binge/purge cycle' is associated with intra-oral manifestations such as lingual erosion of the teeth and bilateral swelling of the parotid glands, and several other common indications outlined in Table 10.2 below.

Another issue of concern relates to eating disorders such as anorexia nervosa and bulimia nervosa or anorexia athletica in female athletes [1,13]. Eating disorders in athletes are further compounded when the female athlete trains excessively. This combination often results in inadequate net caloric intake that can progress to amenorrhea that occurs after menarche. Continued amenorrhea can contribute to the onset of premature osteoporosis with decreased bone mass

Table 10.2 Signs and symptoms that may be included in anorexia athletica.

Fear of weight gain in a lean person	Excess fatigue
Increase in exercise and reduction in food intake	Dehydration
Anxiety	Binge eating
Delayed puberty	Excess use of smokeless tobacco or other methods to suppress appetite
Gastrointestinal complaints	Energy intake below training need

and increased fracture risk. This set of factors (i.e. eating disorder/excessive training, amenorrhea, and osteoporosis) has been termed the 'female athlete triad' [13–16].

Ranalli [13] comments that the 'female athlete triad' throws up many unanswered medical questions [5], such as:

- Is the bone density loss in premature osteoporosis reversible?
- Is premature bone loss in the female athlete triad related to premature alveolar bone loss?

Ranalli [13] calls for continued future research to clarify these issues in relation to female athletes and their optimal care. However the athlete may be hiding their condition from sports coaches or other sports medicine practitioners. Therefore, the dental professional may be the first and only person who identifies any early signs of these conditions, through screening, which can manifest in the female dentition. All these issues must be carefully considered and managed sensitively. The athlete's consent rights to information sharing must be strictly respected. If suspecting a patient is suffering in this way, the sports dentist should seek the help of medical colleagues, to support the athlete.

10.7 Dental Caries

There is evidence to suggest that professional sportspersons have higher caries rates than the equivalent age people in the general population, and that they are at an increased risk of dental erosion, resulting in potentially a greater dental treatment need (see Figure 10.4) [17–29]. This may be due in part to the relatively high carbohydrate and acidic beverage intake used for energy and rehydration during training and playing that has been as alluded to [1–3,5,6,18,28,30].

Poor oral hygiene resulting in plaque deposits, frequent sugar intake, and reduced saliva flow during periods of dehydration, all enhance the bacterial degradation of carbohydrates providing an acidic source for tooth surface demineralisation and carious lesion formation. If left unattended this may rapidly progress to an irreversible cavity that requires restorative intervention.

The dentist should be aware that, in certain endurance sports, such as cycling, long-distance running, and triathlons, the consumption of refined carbohydrates could be very high. As mentioned, these athletes snack regularly to maintain

(a)   (b)

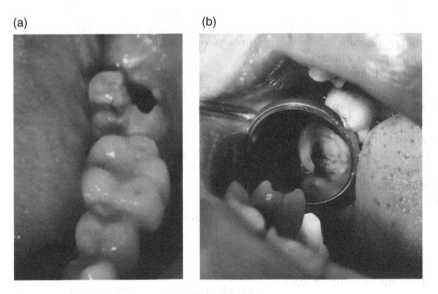

Figure 10.4 Dental caries on tooth LL7 (a) and UL6 (b).

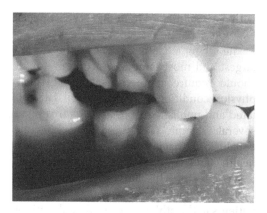

Figure 10.5 Tooth surface loss due to prolonged constant straw holding in between teeth and sipping from an energy drinks bottle in a triathlete.

sufficiently high levels of energy or 'carbo-load' prior to an event. They may also consume sport drinks and carbohydrate gels during competition. Bryant's study on triathletes [18] confirmed these dietary habits, showing frequent high-sugar snack and sports drink intake (Figure 10.5). Worryingly only 3.2% of the athletes in this study were aware and able to associate training and dietary patterns as being of high risk for detriment to their oral health.

Ashley et al. reviewed the literature for evidence of poor oral health in elite sport and concluded that previous studies lacked good comparative or control data.

It is in this author's own previous initial experience in sport when in the infancy of treating professional footballers, that a multitude of dental issues were found. It was discovered that players were attending for emergency dental appointments the day before a game with irreversible pulpitic symptoms or intra-oral/extra-oral swellings. The players would wish a 'quick fix' to the problem to be able to play. Once the initial pain symptoms or swelling had subsided, subsequent appointments were not attended for follow-on care and treatment, as advised to stabilise oral health. Access to players was difficult and no baseline dental records or radiographs were held on the majority of players. Therefore should one of

the club medical staff phone for advice if the team were travelling to away games, it was very difficult to triage the situation. It was also found that players attended with extra-oral swellings due to poor oral health through dental decay, which subsequently impacted and caused a delay to other medical procedures planned for treatment under general anaesthesia. As a result of this and frustration at not being able to provide optimal care and advice, this author decided, with the permission of the club staff, to conduct an initial small pilot dental screen/questionnaire study to assess the scale of the problem. The following key results were noted and the study is unpublished:

- Untreated dental decay in footballers is a problem.
- The 22–25 year age group had the highest rates of decay, with little thought for decay prevention.
- Footballers screened had a higher decayed, missing, filled (DMF) value at (9.09) than the UK Adult Dental Health survey of 2009 (6.9).
- The 26–29 year old age group have had multiple complex dental inventions that could compromise tooth retention long term and post career.
- A match-day dental trauma protocol was only in place for half of the clubs questioned.
- Thirty per cent of professional clubs had ruled out players from matches between one and three times a season due to dental infections.

As a result of this data, the sports medicine department implemented dental health screening as part of their pre-season medical screening in an attempt to gather data and identify 'at-risk' players. This data was also used by the Football Association of England to collate and distribute dental health recommendations to all football league clubs in England in 2014, as outlined below.

10.8   FA Initiative 2014

In recognition of the dental health issues in professional football, the FA Medical Committee released guidance to all professional football clubs in the UK to encourage clubs to adopt the following:

- *Club dentist* – Identify a local dentist for care, including screening/education and dental trauma management.
- *Emergency action plan* – develop and disseminate a plan for training and match day dental trauma management.
- *Funding* – develop clear pathways for funding care, e.g. health partners, stand alone dental insurance (ideally to include sports trauma cover).

The FA utilised the results from this pilot study and drew the following conclusions:

1) Dental decay was not uncommon and was poorly addressed by players.
2) Pre-season and signing medicals may not screen for poor dental health.
3) Preventative care was rare.
4) Emergency dental plans for trauma may or may not be present.
5) Lack of a formal club dentist in many clubs for screening or treating.
6) Uncertainty regarding insurance cover for non-traumatic dental issues and the impact of poor dental health on performance.

Ljungberg's 1990 study within Swedish soccer [23] and Gay-Escoda's 2011 study on FC Barcelona football players [31], illustrated they also had higher DMF scores and mean active carious lesions when compared to students of the same age. Gay-Escoda's study showed, quite surprisingly, that despite repeated dental screening over several seasons, even at an elite football club like FC Barcelona, a multitude of dental issues were presenting for players in season.

The review by Ashley et al. of professional and elite sport shows similar findings across a wide range of sports [17]. Similar findings of high caries rates, oral pain, and poor oral health have also been reported in athletes with disabilities attending the Special Olympics [13,32–37].

The Olympic Games is one of the world's largest and most famous sporting events. It should require competitors to be in peak physical condition. However, dental data collated and published from athletes treated at several Olympic Games all draw the same conclusions, that elite athletes have poor oral health and multiple dental pathologies [28,29,38–40]. This author has seen these issues first hand from time spent treating patients in the athlete's village dental clinic at the London 2012 Olympic and Paralympic games. London 2012 games data from needleman et al. [39] shows high levels of preventable conditions such as dental caries, dental erosion, and periodontal diseases. It was further commented that oral health should be seen as a key determinant of quality of life. Needleman et al. go on to outline that there is a plethora of supporting evidence that poor oral health, symptomatic teeth, and the psychosocial issues associated with dental pain will all impact quality of life [39]. In the London 2012 study, 30% of participants reported on the impact of oral health on their quality of life and nearly 20% on their training or performance.

This author's pilot study results were expanded on and utilized in planning Needleman's 2015 screening study in professional football [41]. Tentative comparisons were made against the 2009 Adult Dental Health Survey (ADHS). Footballers were noted to have higher dentine caries rates in the 16–24 age group (38.3%) compared to 30% in the ADHS. In total, 69.8% of 16–24-year-old footballers, and 88.3% of 25–34-year-olds had one or more restorations. Comparable figures from the ADHS were 53% and 75%. This study was one of the largest single sport dental health studies conducted to date. It has continued to demonstrate and strengthen the evidence base demonstrating high levels of poor oral health and an associated impact among professional footballers. Almost 4 out of 10 players had untreated dental caries. Experience of

(a)

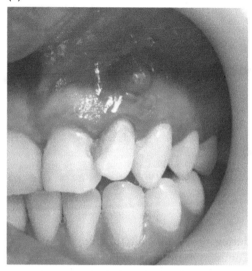

(b)

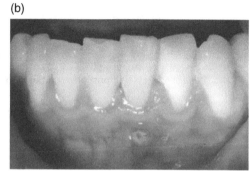

Figure 10.6 Dental (abscess) swelling and chronic infection associated with upper (a) and lower (b) front tooth.

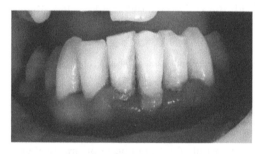

Figure 10.7 Clinical picture of poor oral hygiene with gingival inflammation and calculus.

dental caries or restorations was seen to increase with age. Dental erosion was present in more than half of footballers. Inflammatory gingivitis was seen in over 80% of players and irreversible periodontitis in 5%. Sixteen per cent of players reported current problems or pain in their mouths on presenting to screen. Self-reported impact on health was seen to be significantly associated with dental caries, current dental pain, swellings attributed to wisdom teeth and tooth sensitivity (Figures 10.6–10.8). Almost half of all players (45%) reported to being 'bothered' by their oral health and almost 20% reported it affected their quality of life, with 7% reporting an impact on training or performance.

10.9 Acute and Chronic Infections

10.9.1 Saliva Function

Saliva has a crucial role in tooth protection due to its chemical composition, and the physical and mechanical effects of saliva flow. Saliva aids us in digestion, lubrication, speech, taste, and buffering.

Saliva has a role in dental caries inhibition through:

- Immunological function:
  - Secretory IgA (S-IgA) prevents oral microorganisms adhering to the enamel pellicle
- Enzymatic function:
  - Peroxidase inhibits acid production and reproduction of oral microbes
  - Lysozyme contributes to bacterial cell degradation
- Mechanical function by bathing and cleaning teeth surfaces
- Protective remineralisation of carious lesions through fluoride and calcium ions.

Foster and Readman [42] allude to work by Shinkai et al. (1993) and Rohde et al. (1996)

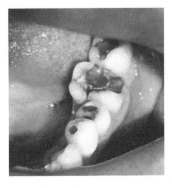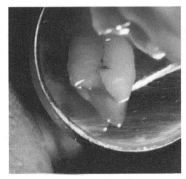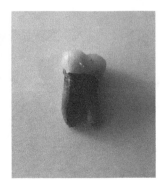

Figure 10.8 Clinical pictures demonstrating cracked tooth syndrome from bruxism.

that identified a relationship between physical stress and exertion and immunosuppression following Olympic-distance triathlon training and competition. D'Ercole et al. [9] and Foster and Redman [42] refer also to a 1999 paper by Gleeson et al., that reported that, compared to before training, a decrease in the concentration of salivary immunoglobin A (IgA) levels are seen in competitive swimmers after training. Secretory IgA (S-IgA) is the main immunoglobulin found in defense against oral pathogens.

These combined findings represent a small but significant window for post-training and -competition athlete immunosuppression. D'Ercole et al. [9] reportede several studies linking this to an increased incidence of upper respiratory tract infections in sportspeople. Therefore IgA appears to act as a marker for mucosal immunity and its decreased levels specifically sampled from the mouth can predict possible negative effects on general health and wellbeing. However, D'Ercole et al further comment that these findings conflict with other authors who state that there are no differences in salivary concentrations of S-IgA between athletes and non-athletes, except when athletes are engaged in excessive heavy training volumes.

Therefore, previously asymptomatic and potentially underlying chronic oral conditions can manifest with an acute clinical symptoms

during times of bodily immunosuppression. Common examples can include pericoronitis associated to partially erupted wisdom teeth and chronic periapical dental lesions associated with non-vital teeth. In an acute phase, both may disrupt the training nutritional needs and performance of the athlete.

10.9.2 Third Molars (Wisdom Teeth) and Pericoronitis

Pericoronitis is the inflammation of the operculum (flap of gingival tissue around a partially erupted tooth). It is combinative result of food and plaque trapping, poor oral hygiene, or mechanical trauma. It is commonly associated to the third molars and presents mainly in the late teens and early twenties.

Commonly the gingival tissue around the tooth is painful and swollen with a potential foul taste in the mouth from purulent discharge. The athlete may complain about the difficulty and restrictions in opening wide (trismus). Further extra-oral symptoms can include lymphadenopathy and swelling. Debridement of any food packing around the gingival tissue may need to be undertaken in conjunction with chlorhexidine or hot saltwater mouth rinses. Sometimes antibiotics are required with acute symptoms.

Pericoronitis in an athlete can compromise nutrition, training, and competition schedules. Therefore early recognition and assessment of third molar status and adequate oral hygiene instruction are essential around partially erupted teeth.

10.10 Temporomandibular Joint Dysfunction

Foster and Readman allude to Beaton's 1991 paper, suggesting stress may manifest itself as temporomandibular joint dysfunction [42]. Extra-oral examination and occlusal analysis for signs of attritive wear facets should form part of any screening examination. Athletes should be questioned on temporomandibular joint dysfunction symptoms, previous history, and any associated trauma. Bruxism diagnosis may require fabrication of an occlusal splint to prevent an acute episode of pain. It maybe prudent that any study casts used in either an occlusal splint or a mouth guard fabrication could be duplicated and retained. These casts can then be kept as a hard record of the dentition for ongoing monitoring of the rate of tooth surface loss.

10.11 Barotrauma

10.11.1 Barodontaligia

This is termed oral pain, caused by changes in barometric pressure. It can occur during flying, diving, mountain climbing, and in hyperbaric chambers or other environmental pressure scenarios. In-flight barodontalgia is reported at altitudes as low as 2000 feet and as high as 35 000 feet, but it is more common between 9000 and 27 000 feet [43].

During diving, barodontalgia may occur at a water depth of 33–86 feet [18]. However, during flying, theoretically possible pressure changes range from 1 atmosphere (at ground level) to 0 atmosphere (at outer space); the changes are more significant during diving because each descent of 10 m (32.8 feet) elevates the pressure by 1 atmosphere [44].

Table 10.3 Zadik's [45] summary of Frejentsik and Aker (1982) barotrauma classification.

Class	Cause	Symptoms
I	Non-reversible pulpitis	Sharp pain on ascent
II	Reversible pulpitis	Dull throbbing pain on ascent
III	Necrotic pulp	Dull throbbing pain on decent
IV	Periapical lesions	Severe persistent pain on ascent and decent

Excellent summary papers by Robichaud and McNally [46] and Zadik [45] (Table 10.3) reflected that most of the existing barotrauma evidence has been sourced from military medicine. Incidences of in-flight dental manifestations as a result of pressure changes are low. It was reported that between 2.4 and 8.2%, and up to half of 499 Spanish, 331 Israeli, and 135 Saudi Arabian and Kuwaiti Air Force aircrews reported at least one episode of barodontalgia. Interestingly, it is thought that this low occurrence rate is due to current low pressurisation of aeroplane cabins, pilots having high-quality dental care, and the improvement of oral health in the second half of the twentieth century. By comparison, could the same be said of our current sportspeople, considering the current evidence of poor oral health?

Currently, there is no definitive consensus on the pathogenesis of pulp-related barodontalgia. However, a healthy pulp appears to be unaffected by barometric change. It is suggested that when divers submerge, inspired air may enter a tooth under pressure via structural defects such as carious cavities, defective restorations, cracks, or less commonly gas dissolved in pulpal blood vessels. It is believed this is more likely to happen in the presence of hyperemic tissues. Pain is therefore due to trapped air expansion in a rapidly changing pressure environment. As a result air is forced into tooth dental tubules, which in turn stimulates pain fibers [43,44,46,47].

In endodontically treated teeth, pain may be associated with trapped air bubble expansion within or under the root filling. In teeth with associated periapical periodontitis, pain symptoms are most likely due to a heightening in pressure within the bony periapical lesion.

Jagger et al. [47], Kini et al. [43], Robichaud and McNally [46], and Zadik [44] all report that recent restorative treatment was reported as a major cause of symptoms. Patients in an acute inflammatory phase or with infection should not fly, as pressure changes could cause spread of infection or recent extraction sites could be prone to secondary hemorrhaging and pain. A suggested 'no fly' time period of between 24 and 72 hours post treatment is an effective means for preventing post-operative barodontalgia or seven days is advised following surgery. In respect of this, any dental treatment should be planned in advance of the next planned flight or dive.

Kini et al. [43], Robichaud and McNally [46], and Zadik [44] outline that prevention of barodontalgia, relies on good oral health and periodic dental screening. Defective (fractured or cracked) restorations, restorations with poor retention, and secondary caries lesions should be noted and treated. Pulp testing and periapical radiographs should be performed in teeth with pre-existing extensive restorations to rule out undiganosed pulp necrosis. It is suggested that panoramic radiographs at three to five year intervals for people at a higher risk for barodontalgia should be undertaken. Jagger et al. [47] allude to compulsory annual medical examinations by the Health and Safety Executive (HSE) (MA1) [48] medical staff for professional divers to be certified of a high standard of physical health to dive. This encourages dental screening and regular dental examinations, a high standard of dental care and a certification of dental fitness also, which is very encouraging.

This unusual phenomenon requires consideration in modern day sport. Many long distances may be travelled for international competitions and also short flights nationally to avoid long bus journeys. The use of hyperbaric oxygen therapy may also be required for treatment of certain conditions and a healthy dentition is essential and should not limit or prohibit treatment.

10.12 Mouth Guards

Dental trauma prevention and other sporting injuries have become an even more important issue owing to an increased popularity of contact sport at a young age.

A mouth guard is a key feature in dental trauma impact minimisation and prevention of orofacial injuries (Figure 10.9). The team dentist must supply players with a proper, well-fitting guard and be able to provide the appropriate education to players, sports medics, coaches, and parents on the benefits of the sometimes confusing plethora of mouth guards available on the market. As dental health professionals, we should be encouraging their use at all levels of sport.

Newsome, Owen, and Read [35] refer toDorney's 1998 study of elite Australian rugby players' oral health and mouth guard use, and from direct discussion with the author, determined traumatic dental injury rates were seen in one in two players. None of the players' mouth guards inspected at screening were satisfactory. There was a multitude of untreated dental decay and dental erosion. An increase in the incidence of sports drinks sponsorships and therefore player uptake, potentially contributes to being a causative factor in high caries rates.

Mouth guard programmess should be organised and run in conjunction with a team dental screening or organised and planned from the data collected from the dental screen. Ideally, sportspeople should be dentally stable and fit, before mouth guard impressions are taken. This will avoid repeated impressions and study cast discrepancies, and paucity of mouth guard fit and retention.

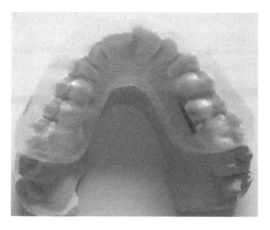 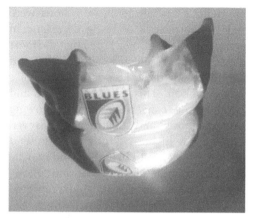

Figure 10.9 Custom-made mouth guards fabricated on a dental model taken from an accurate impression.

Appropriate mouth guard recommendations can be made relative to the type of sport and level of competition. It is outside the scope of this chapter to fully discuss mouth guards and this is covered further in Chapter 7.

10.13   Other Issues

Several fashionable habits in society are reflected in sports men and women [14]. These may include various forms of tattoos and intra-oral piercings. Ranalli outlines dental literature regarding adverse intra-oral and systemic effects in relation to tongue and lip piercings, namely fractured teeth and gingival stripping [13].

10.13.1   Snus

Another issue of growing concern relates to the use of smokeless tobacco in sportspersons. Needleman et al. [41] found that 5.4% of professional footballers screened were using Snus (a moist powder tobacco pouch; Figure 10.10), which is of concern and previously unheard of. Screening for oral cancer and early recognition of potential dysplastic oral soft tissue lesions has been common practice for many years. There are several reports of a rising worldwide incidence of oral cancer, with recent trends for a rising

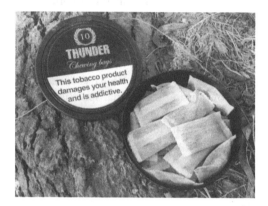

Figure 10.10 Snus.

incidence of tongue and mouth cancer in young males. Most studies suggest that 4–6% of oral cancers now occur at ages younger than 40 years. Several studies examining risk factors for oral cancer in the young provide evidence that many younger patients have never smoked or consumed alcohol, which are recognised risk factors in older groups, or that duration of exposure may be too short for malignant transformation to occur [49].

Epstein et al. [50] reported on oral cancer screening to identify early soft tissue lesions, alluding to a 1986 Bouquet and Gorlin study that found the majority of soft tissue lesions showing a change in colour, texture, size, and contour were benign. However, around 17% were oral leukoplakia and 7% were severely dysplastic carcinomas. Sciubba et al. [51]

reported 12% of all epithelial lesions were clinically suspicious of being dysplastic in nature. Epstein et al. concluded that the most effective way to decrease morbidity and mortality with these lesions is to increase early detection. This involves baseline and repeated oral cancer screenings, allowing early diagnosis and treatment. However, people in the higher-risk groups often tend to have poorer health behaviors and may be less likely to undergo screening and follow-on care. A randomized trial in India reported that oral screening was followed by a 34% reduction in oral cancer mortality among users of tobacco or alcohol or both, and a much higher reduction in those complying with all rounds of screening.

Oral health questionnaires can provide an insight and indication on lifestyle habits (e.g. nutritional) beyond notoriously inaccurate self-reporting. The increasing use of chewing tobacco/Snus in professional sport is worrying. Dentists should introduce oral cancer screening, to include extensive soft tissue examination and questioning on tobacco habits, as good practice when forming screening protocols.

10.14 Sports Team Dentist Roles and Responsibilities

Many sports teams or clubs may or may not have an associated team dentist, who can form part of a larger and wider professional sports medicine team and club staff who will be responsible for the total care and conditioning of the athlete. It is essential that good lines of communication and mutual role appreciation exist within and between all team members of the sports medicine team for a harmonious and productive relationship.

In consideration of the International Academy for Sports Dentistry guidance the following highlight the key roles, attributes, and responsibilities a dentist should be able to bring to a sports medicine team:

- Organise pre-season screening. Treat and coordinate dental care for the team athletes and players. This ensures all are dentally healthy for the start of a competitive season.
- Work within a multi-disciplinary (non-dental) team. Be able to discuss and contribute at player management meetings with sports medicine staff.
- Be confident and have the appropriate knowledge, experience, and skill in immediate dental and orofacial trauma management.
- Establish an emergency dental trauma management protocol for match and competition days.
- Have the appropriate dental knowledge on common acute and chronic conditions that may be sports related and advise on treatment and management in respect to the athletes training and competing ability.
- Establish and supply the required dental equipment for emergency management on match/competition days if covering an event.
- Adequate level of training. Possess the knowledge to work within clinical experience boundaries. If outside those boundaries, then be able to have the appropriate list of available contacts with specialist skills for onward prompt referral.
- Maintain accurate dental records be it computerised or safe/secure storage of hard paper copies.
- Provide immediate emergency dental care in respect of the athlete's availability and training playing /competing schedule.
- Consider prevention of dental trauma for those athletes/players that have a higher predisposition to traumatic dental injuries. This may take the form of instigating club/team mouth guard programmes.
- Provide adequate education on oral hygiene advice to athletes and club team staff.
- Provision of continued professional development training and education on dental topics in relation to sport.
- Ensure the appropriate indemnity cover is in place.

- Protection of the player/athlete, who is the sport dentist's patient and respecting his or her confidentiality at all times in relation to requests for information from outside sources/club team staff.

Kumamoto [52] outlined that the three most important criteria out of all the above listed responsibilities are the provision of pre-season screening, rapid emergency dental care, and the education and supply of mouth guards for dental trauma prevention.

10.15 Screening Programmes

General medical screening programmes usually involve large groups of a seemingly healthy population undergoing testing with a simple, easy-to-use, acceptable, and affordable screening test. The main rationale for screening is to identify members of the public likely to have a particular disease and to either confirm or exclude the disease. Most people may choose to be screened, to be reassured that they are healthy. Early screening for cancer aims at providing early recognition of pre-cancerous lesions. This allows effective early treatment to prevent death from an invasive cancer and to improve the quality of life.

In planning a screening programme, the ability to offer further investigation for those showing a positive test, treatment, and follow-on care of those diagnosed with disease must be thought out. Screening programmes should be subject to quality assurance, constant review, and evaluation of the service.

The advantages and disadvantages of screening are outlined in Table 10.5.

The ability to introduce screening programmes may differ significantly between high-, middle-, and low-income countries. The under-developed health services and lack of resources precludes the introduction of screening programmes in many low-income countries.

The same can be said of sports teams or clubs. Annual club or sports medicine budget constraints may restrict the ability to introduce dental health screening programs.

As this author has demonstrated previously in professional football, the introduction of pilot programmes prior to escalation to a full screening program across multiple players or squads has proved beneficial in supporting athletes. It aids the dental professional in controlling the screening process and highlights the results and benefits to sports medicine staff if it were to be applied across multiple teams/squads, nationally and internationally.

10.15.1 Barriers to Dental Care

In establishing a dental screening programme within sport and subsequently attempting to organize follow-on care, several hurdles frequently need to be overcome to avoid restriction to care compared to the 'normal' dental patient (Table 10.4). As has been anecdotally reported by this author's experiences, athletes are poor dental attenders, only seeking advice when a dental issue arises. Athletes are also superstitious regarding proposed treatment in season or near a competition. An attitude of 'if it's not hurting why treat it' is frequently encountered rather than accepting a preventative approach.

Several other restrictive factors include:

- Training sessions over-running and unscheduled extra sessions
- Dental practice opening hours
- Travel (nationally and internationally)
- Other medical treatments (physiotherapy/surgery)
- Individual or team meetings
- Media commitments
- Dental phobia (never had a dental visit previously)
- Huge personalities or egos
- May not book the appointments – agent / PA/ club secretaries
- School work
- Cost, depending on level competing at and available salary.

Table 10.4 The advantages/disadvantages and considerations of screening.

Advantages of screening	Disadvantages of screening
Disease is suitable to screen and a straightforward predictable test exists	Over-diagnosis and over-treatment
High level of quality evidence, demonstrated by screening morbidity is reduced	Wasted resources
Screening benefits outweigh any potential physical and psychological detriment resultant of testing, diagnosis, and treatment.	Unconsidered complications by intervening/participant anxiety
Adequate human and financial resources to provide the screen and accessible follow-up treatment	Organised Uptake on follow-on care post screen
Cost-effectiveness and cost-benefit analyses carried out Appropriate information to enable valid informed consent for all participants	Cost
Need and drive and willingness for the introduction of the screening programme	High participation and compliance

10.15.2 Objectives of Dental Screening

With regards to a dental screen, the objectives within sport can be further broken down (Table 10.5).

Callaghan and Jarvis's 1986 paper [19] outlined the British Cycling Federation (BCF) establishment of their medical screening for international elite riders. This was undertaken in the winter off-season to obtain early diagnoses of hidden pathologies and monitor 'known' medical conditions. It was felt important that all medical practitioners had previous involvement within cycling, and were familiar with examination and management

Table 10.5 Objectives of dental screening.

Detect underlying conditions that would hamper or limit athlete participation

Identify previous dental problems and potential short / long term problems

Establish a baseline record of general dental health to allow building of an athlete or player career dental portfolio

Establish a squad/team database and identify those higher risk athletes who require treatment and further investigation

Injury prevention policy – inspection and supply of mouth guards

of professional cyclists. Callaghan and Jarvis commented that personnel familiar and interested in the sport aided the smooth running of the screening programme, enhanced communication between professions, and minimised disruption during the medical screening process. They concluded that the squad medical screen is important to assess elite cyclists. It demonstrated that a structured system could help early diagnosis and treatment to provide injury-free cyclists in readiness for the start of a competitive season.

Dental examination revealed 21% of cyclists needed follow-on care. Despite issues being flagged in the 1991 pre-season three cyclists returned in 1992 with the same issue, and had failed to seek treatment. It was commented further that a number of cyclists had a dental phobia and completely avoided the free dental screen available.

In the armed services, the following risk dental assessment categories have been used for many years. Richardson [43,53] outlined that personnel were classified according to the following 'NATO standard agreement 2466' categories:

1) Full dentally fit.
2) Dental treatment required, but the condition is not expected to cause a problem in the next year.

3) Treatment is required and the condition is expected to cause problems within the next year.

4) Dental examination overdue.

Only service personnel in categories 1 and 2 were deployed on duty. Despite this, several studies by Allen and Smith (1992), McClave and Brokaw (1988) and Grover et al. (1983) reported that in personnel from category 3, between 34% and 85% went on to develop dental symptoms within 12 months [53,54]. Interestingly Allen and Smith/Chaffin et al. (2001) and Mahoney and Combs (2000) reported dental morbidity rates of approximately 150–160 personnel per 1000, even when no category 3 troops were deployed. It was commented that several dental scenarios are completely unpredictable, such as restorations fracturing, a loss of tooth vitality without any prior signs, or a person sustaining a traumatic dental injury.

Richardson's 2005 paper [54] went on to outline that UK armed forces have now use a high, medium, and low dental risk categorization. It is interesting to note that British army personnel have always had poorer oral health than the RAF and royal navy personnel. This is attributed to the variation in the socio-demographic profiles of the recruits between the respective services. Such is the worldwide popularity of sports participation that this statement may also be true in the sporting world. As has been demonstrated in studies during the Olympic Games and professional football, athletes may come into elite training programmes or sports clubs from a variety of socioeconomic backgrounds and cultures. Richardson concludes that it is totally impossible to prevent dental morbidity, but that there is scope to reduce morbidity rates up to 25% by ensuring all personnel are as dentally fit as feasible by regular screening.

10.15.3 Dental Screening Practicalities

Routine pre-season/pre-competition screening may not take place in the dental surgery (Figure 10.11), but at a team/club training

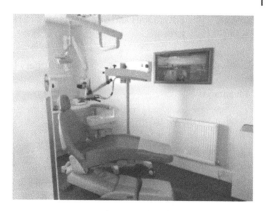

Figure 10.11 Typical dental surgery for optimal dental examination.

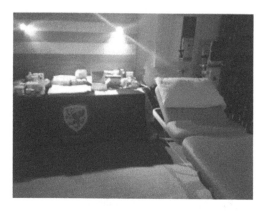

Figure 10.12 Off-site dental screening facility will vary according to circumstances.

base or ground (Figure 10.12). The dental staff undertaking the screening process may therefore be outside their own normal clinical comfort zone in working within the limited facilities available. Therefore, prior preparation and readiness are the two main factors in organizing a dental pre-season screening session to maximize productivity. The varying advantages and disadvantages of a dental-surgery based screen or on-site training-based facility screen are outlined in Table 10.6. The screening dental professional may wish to consider the practicalities of these points. An open discussion should be undertaken with the associated sports medicine staff on the facilities available should the screen be off-site from the dental surgery, and the dental limitations associated to this.

Table 10.6 The advantages and disadvantages of a dental surgery-based screening program vs. an on-site training facility screen.

Dental surgery-based screen	
Advantages	**Disadvantages**
Familiar surroundings for dental staff	Athlete/player may not have dentist to present to for a dental examination
Continuity of care and dedicated dental computerised records available	Athletes/players may have limited time to attend appointments
Opportunity to have time for a complete dental appointment with no other athlete distractions	Varying knowledge of dental staff on sports issues depending on experience and advice given
No equipment restrictions and full range available (radiographs and good light source)	Cost
Support staff nurse reception / hygiene	Attendance issues (failed to attend, last minute cancellations, turning up late in a busy dental appointment list)
Access and the ability to undertake on the day urgent care or temporary dressings if time allows	Lack of immediate communication with club staff

On-site training facility screen	
Advantages	**Disadvantages**
Specialist knowledgeable personnel	Noisy, hurried, disorganised
Efficient, cost-effective	Lack of privacy
Direct communication club staff on the day	Difficulty in follow-up and lack of communication from parents of younger athletes
Direct access to players and athletes	Appropriate record keeping
If properly organised can work well around training and players down time	Lack of materials, i.e. dental chair/radiographs inappropriate light source
Easier for club/team to organise as part of general preseason screening day	Other commitments restrict time
	On the day change of circumstances (absent athletes /players)

Of the papers sourced as outlined, comparisons of screening methods can be drawn between screening of military personnel ready for deployment and sportspeople. The benefits of oral cancer screening have also been highlighted. Needleman et al. [55] commented that in accordance with the Wilson and Jungner screening criteria, the screening of oral health seems fully justified within football and sport, given the high prevalence of treatable conditions being seen from dental health studies.

10.15.4 Pre-season Screening

This author has mainly undertaken sports training facility-based screens. If properly organized and set up, this can run very effectively for a quick basic visual dental assessment. Each athlete or player can then be prioritised and recalled to the dental surgery for further investigation based on the screening data collated. Should the screen be undertaken off-site, it is also useful to liaise with the sports medicine team to organise a list of timings for the players to present for screening.

This dental screen may form part of medical pre-season screening rotation day. Again, from this author's experience, most athletes are allocated and seen at 15–20 minute intervals. To maximise the consultation time there must be adequate time set aside for newer squad members to build a relationship.

Depending on the number of dental staff available and the number of athletes or players requested to be screened, this can be carried out over two days, if required. The important fact to consider and remember is that this dental screening process must fit in and around the sportspersons' daily commitments and other sports medicine practitioners' treatments or investigations. The aim is to avoid minimal interruption to their daily schedule. From this author's discussions with sports medicine practitioners, general pre-season medical screening of athletes is suggested to be undertaken four to eight weeks before the start of a competitive season. A dental screening programme should run parallel to this, either independently or as part of a planned medical general screening day or days. This will also allow adequate time to carry out the necessary treatment pre-season/pre-competition or pre-tour. Mandatory screening should be carried out at least once a season, if not twice if time allows.

It is prudent at the start of the screening process to undertake informed consent with the player or athlete. An example of several consent questions to consider may include the following:

1) *I give my consent to a dental examination and understand this is for the purpose of outlining a brief assessment of my dental health status.*

   I agree   I disagree

2) *I give my consent to discuss the findings of this dental examination with the sports medicine department of .... to formulate a future dental care plan*

   I agree   I disagree

3) *I give my consent for the anonymous use of any dental photographs for publication and education purposes and my full name or face will never be used in these and I cannot be identified*

   I agree   I disagree

4) *I give my consent for the anonymous use of clinical data gathered from this dental screen for education and research purposes and my full name shall never be used and I cannot be identified by this data*

   I agree   I disagree

A suggested basic list of instruments/disposables and materials for an off-site screening session or mouth guard session is summarised in Table 10.7.

An example of a typical screening proforma/dental examination sheet is shown below.

Table 10.7 Dental materials list.

Gloves	Alginate	Periodontal probes
Masks	Mixing bowl	Spare box for impressions
Loupes / light source	Spatula	Sharps boxes
Bibs	Measuring scoops	Clinical waste bags
Stationary (pens stapler)	Steri -wipes	Additional dental staff
Data screening sheets	Impression trays of varying sizes	Cotton rolls / pledgets
Hand gels	Ribbon wax	Tweezers
Sticky labels	Mouth mirrors	Verify numbers for screening session
Clear bags	Gauze	Squad list / staff and timings
Paper towels	Disposable exam kits	Time frame for screening

The screen maybe include two components: a player questionnaire and the examination.

1) *Questionnaire:* The player questionnaire should question how regular is dental attendance, dental issues within the last twelve months, tobacco use, sports drink use, oral health regimes.

2) *Examination:* Like any dental examination, the dental screen should involve a comprehensive past dental history taking and through clinical examination:

- Presenting complaint
- History presenting complaint
- Past dental history (to include dental trauma history)
- Medical history
- Social history
- Extra oral examination (to include):
  - TMJ
  - Muscles of mastication palpation
  - Lymph node palpation
- Intra-oral examination (to include):
  - Soft tissue exam
  - Dental chart of teeth present and dental status (3rd molar status)
  - Dental caries/defective restorations (decayed/missing/filled)
  - Oral health and periodontal status (BPE)
  - Occlusal analysis and jaw relations
- Current mouth guard status, if applicable, and examination.

After screening completion the dental professional will need to collate the data and identify the 'at risk athletes and dentitions'. In Table 10.8 caries risk assessment factors are highlighted that should be considered when trying to categorise players' risk [56,57]. Historically, players have been commonly categorized as high-, medium- or low-risk for dental symptoms and treatment priority.

As long as a player's consent is gained, this information can then be shared with the associated sports medicine department, and an individual player and squad breakdown on dental status can be given. Player confidentiality should be respected and

Table 10.8 The important factors in caries assessment.

The number of active lesions that are cavitated or non-cavitated
The history of new lesions filled in the past two to three years and how many lesions are present
Multiple active lesions in areas of rapid salivary flow (lower incisor and buccal surface of molars shows high caries activity)
A yearly increment of two or more lesions indicates a high rate of lesion activity and progression
An athlete who may consume a high carbohydrate diet before, during, and after exercise, in addition to transitional meals, is classed as a high caries risk.

maintained if consent is refused to screen or release data. Examples of a screening examination and subsequent player report sheet are included in Figures 10.13 & 10.14 that this author has constructed, adopted, and changed over several previous sports dental screens.

It is in this author's experience that, despite flagging problems to the player or sports medicine department, it can be difficult to work through the screened squad list fully to convert all higher- or medium-risk athletes to a low-risk category. Screening is being seen as important, yet the follow-up of dental treatment can be seen as a low priority. It is often left to the athlete or player to attend the dental practice and the barriers to care previously mentioned prove problematic. This author feels at present as a sports medicine profession this is an area in which there is a breakdown. Considering the initial objectives of introducing a screening programme, further efforts must be made to follow up on players who have undergone screening to re-emphasise the need to follow the screening and subsequent treatment process through.

However, this author again has found that it can be very difficult to persuade sportspeeople to attend for treatment, when they may not perceive there is a problem or not have any pain. As with the 'normal day to day' dental patient, compliance will depend

PRE-SEASON DENTAL HEALTH SCREENING QUESTIONNAIRE

Please complete all sections on pages 1 and 2 below and tick or circle.

Name: Date of Birth:

- **When did you last have a dental check up?**
  0–3 months,   3–6 months,   6–9 months,   9–12 months,   12 months +
- **Do you currently have your own local dentist?**
  Y / N
- **Are you anxious about having dental treatment: -**
  Y / N
- **Do you currently use any form of tobacco or Snus?**
- Y / N
- **Do you have any dental problems or pain in your mouth at the moment?**
  Y / N
- **Have you had any dental pain or problems within the last 12 months?**
  Y / N
- **Have you ever had to miss any training or games due to a dental problem?**
  Y / N
- **Have you ever had any swelling or infections around your wisdom teeth?**
  Y / N
- **How often on average per week do you use sports drinks?**
  Don't use,   1–2 times ,   3–5 times ,   6+ times a week
- **Have you had any dental or jaw injuries to your teeth from playing football?**
  Y/ N

(Please answer all questions 1–4 and circle the answers)

1. I give my consent to a dental examination and understand this is for the purpose to outline a brief assessment of my dental health status.

I agree   I disagree

2. I give my consent to discuss the findings of this dental examination with the .... Sports Medicine Department to formulate a future dental care plan.

I agree   I disagree

3. I give my consent for the anonymous use of any dental photographs for publication and education purposes and my full name or face will never be used.

I agree   I disagree

4. I give my consent for the anonymous use of data gathered from this dental screen for education and research purposes and my full name shall never be used.

I agree   I disagree

SIGNED: **DATE:**

Figure 10.13 A screening examination sheet.

on the patient's personality and attitude to their wellbeing and the importance they place on this.

Through dental screening, the issue of poor oral health and dental issues can be brought to the fore. However, changing attitudes and health/dental behaviours can be very difficult to achieve.

Greenberg et al. [57] allude to Weinstein's adoption process model of changing behavior.

PRE-SEASON DENTAL HEALTH SCREENING EXAMINATION
(DENTIST TO COMPLETE)
BPE

CALCULUS: None   Little   Moderate   Heavy

ORAL HYGIENE: Excellent   Good   Fair   Poor

DENTAL CHARTING

Please include full dental chart any detected or suspected caries. Crown and bridge work, wisdom teeth (fully erupted or partially erupted)

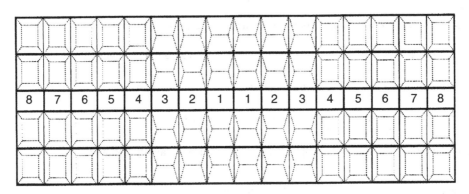

Number of teeth present:

Number of teeth with enamel caries:

Number of teeth with dentine caries:

SOFT TISSUE EXAMINATION

(Unhealthy scored as red / white patches, or ulceration presence)

Mucosal health: healthy   unhealthy

EROSIVE WEAR SCORE

(Please chart worst score for combined upper and lower teeth)

Dental erosion: Anterior teeth: Enamel only   Into Dentine

Dental erosion: Posterior teeth: Enamel only   Into Dentine

SINUSES/SWELLINGS   **Y/ N**

If yes chart adjacent tooth area:

OCCLUSION CLASS: 1   2 (I II)   3

OTHER NOTES: TMJ / 3RD MOLARS /TSL

CARIES STATUS :   High   Medium   Low

TREATMENT NEED PRIORITY: High   Medium   Low

EXAMINED BY / SIGNATURE / DATE

Figure 10.13 (Cont'd)

This proposes that change is best accomplished in seven stages, gradually over time.

1) Patient unaware of the issue
2) Patient unengaged on the issue
3) Patient deciding about action
4) Deciding to act, but not yet in action
5) Deciding not to act
6) Acting
7) Maintenance.

This theory suggests that an individual's beliefs and perceptions about their health maybe a critical element in changing their behaviours. Routine dental screening in sport may facilitate the ultimate goal to adopt a new behaviour or change an existing one. This model maybe implemented into repeated screening of dental non-attenders for care. It should intend to inform sportspeeople about the increased risk of dental symptoms in season, potentially resulting in missing training, competition, or games. Optimistically this may be the jolt needed to move athletes from being unaware and unengaged to becoming aware and engaging in change and undertaking the necessary dental treatment.

If an athlete has been identified as 'at risk' then the dentist should take the necessary steps to minimise the potential damage to the dentition. This may involve a dietary analysis or speaking to the team dietitian. The clinician should be cautious when suggesting changes to the dietary habits of an elite athlete, as this may be strictly regulated. Dental recall appointments should be scheduled more frequently. Early caries remineralisation and caries prevention therapy also has its proven benefits, through the use of high-fluoride dentifrices, mouth rinses, and gels [2,21,56,57,59–62].

As dental professionals, we may need to adopt a slightly different approach to dental care when treating the athlete. The timing of dental treatment or dental pathologies may hinder an athlete's specific sports diet/regime or hydration programme as set out by their nutritionist or participation in their chosen sport. Any post-treatment anesthesia, swelling or trismus as a result of a dental abscess/pericoronitis, or toothache will also influence nutrition or perhaps even other medical treatments and procedures that are required under general anesthesia.

It is therefore imperative that there are good lines of communication between the dental practitioner, the athlete, and the appropriate sports medicine/team personnel. This will establish an athlete/player dental rapport and relationship. A baseline dental portfolio can be assembled and this can be kept with the athlete's or player's medical records, being updated periodically. This can sometimes be difficult for certain sports, such as football players, who can be very transient in nature, or athletics/cycling where overseas training camps and competitions are commonplace, with no access to dental care. Most elite sports medicine practitioners now use specific notation software to allow interaction between various personnel and club staff. It allows the sports medicine team who are responsible for the day-to-day care of that athlete to be more informed. This also leaves nothing to chance or cause a last minute 'dental surprise' when access to dental care maybe problematic. Should a dental issue arise with a 'known' athlete or player then at least the dentist can advise the sports medic appropriately on acute management until attendance at the dental surgery is possible.

Figure 10.14 shows the allied dental healthcare professional network that the team dentist should have in his or her contact armory to allow appropriate onward care for specific scenarios if required post screening.

10.16 Prescribing

As dental healthcare professionals we also need to be wary in our prescription and drug advice to sportspeople who may be under the scrutiny of regular drug testing. Certain drugs can be checked for their prohibition status on the UK and World Antidoping

**FA|WALES
CBD|CYMRU**

Dear Medical Colleague,

As part of the Welsh football Association (WFA) pre-season medical preparations,

.... underwent a basic dental screening examination.

This report can be utilised for the clubs medical team information on their player's dental health. It can also be utilised to liaise with the club or players dentist for treatment planning purposes.
To secure dental health, we would be extremely grateful if you could arrange for investigation of the teeth noted below. This is in the hope of preventing any dental issues during the forthcoming European Championships.

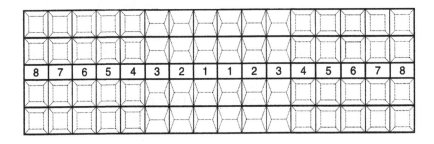

PAST DENTAL HISTORY

CURRENT DENTAL ISSUES /SYMPTOMS

LAST DENTAL VISIT

WISDOM TEETH STATUS

DENTAL TRAUMA HISTORY

1

Figure 10.14 A screening report sheet.

**FA|WALES
CBD|CYMRU**

TOOTHWEAR STATUS

OTHER COMMENTS

SUGGESTED TREATMENT SUMMARY

Scale & polish Oral hygiene, Diet advice sports drinks use. High Fluoride toothpastes and mouthwash advice use	
Radiographic Investigation	
Restorations	
Extractions	
Other Pathology / comments	

If you require any further detailed information about the above-suggested treatment, or if you have any general queries about our screening programme, please do not hesitate to contact me directly via e-mail or phone.

TO THE TREATING DENTIST

Should you feel there is any other on-going dental issues, in which the WFA medical staff should be aware of, please add any additional notes below.

....
....
....
....

2

Figure 10.14 (Cont'd)

FA|WALES
CBD|CYMRU

Once the player is deemed as dentally fit and had all outstanding treatment investigated and completed, we would be grateful if you could sign this form below and return with the player to the WFA medical staff.

Dentists name: ....Date:...........................

Signed:...

Practice address: ....

....
....
....

Thank you in advance for your help. We appreciate you taking the time to help this player achieve dental fitness.

Kind regards,

Mr Lyndon Meehan BDS (Wales), BSc, MJDF RCS (Eng.), MSc Endo
(Dentist to Cardiff City Football Club, Welsh Football Association and Welsh Rugby Union)[1]
Lynddent@yahoo.co.uk

---

[1]Lyndon Meehan and The Welsh Football Association hold the ownership of this confidential document

3

Figure 10.14 (Cont'd)

Agency websites (www.globaldro.com/uk-en, www.wada-ama.org) before recommendation. Again, it may be prudent to document clearly in the patient's records any advice given and any online reference numbers obtained for checks. Liaison with any club medical staff on prescriptions given is essential to avoid overlapping administration.

10.17 Prevention and Considerations for Care

From this author's personal experience in working at international competitions and on discussion with other sports medicine staff, it has been found that in the majority of cases, recognition of a dental issue only occurs when a player or athlete presents to competition or in-season.

Without appropriate education, intervention, and prevention, an athlete may not be aware of the potential dental destruction that may be quiescently ongoing in their mouth until too late. Dental health and attendance tends also be a low priority for athletes and associated staff until a problem arises. Toothache at the wrong moment can sacrifice years or months of training and preparation for competition time. For those athletes who do present for treatment, careful consideration may have to be given to how appointments are scheduled. Athletes may also decline treatment days before competition for mental fear of problems post dental visit. Over the course of a season or a career compromises to the ideal definitive care sometimes must be made to allow for very busy training and competing schedules. The dentist will have to tailor treatment to fit the athlete's needs, lifestyle, and timescales.

Therefore, it is imperative that athletes either undergo or attend for routine periodic dental examinations. Relatively minor and simple dental problems that are left untreated, and that the athlete and sports medicine team are unaware of, could potentially manifest at a crucial later stage as a condition that may completely decimate an athlete's dietary and training regime, or even force him or her to miss competition.

Medical screening of elite sportspeople can be costly and logistically difficult. This can be especially problematic in individual-based sports, which involve a large volume of solo training, and competition times are not in large team squads. In certain off-season periods, athletes in these months can spend little time in contact with elite coaching or medical staff, Consequently, sportspeople can develop problems that may only come to light at the start of the competition process season.

In order to address these issues within sport, a system of periodic dental screening should be established and strongly encouraged (Figure 10.15). The aims of any screening should be to obtain early diagnosis and monitoring of known problems and to diagnose silent diseases. This should also embrace dietary and optimal oral health advice in conjunction with and respective of the athletes dietary and nutritional needs. Therefore it is essential that athletes are screened and declared dentally fit in an off-season period. This will attempt to avoid the need for dental treatment in season.

There is a paucity of high-quality published literature regarding dental screening in sport. This may be attributed to the fact that sports medicine, and sports dentistry in particular,

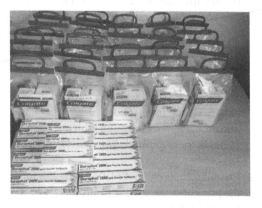

Figure 10.15 A dental screening day is a good time to educate on optimal oral health measures and distribute oral health packs as above.

is a rapidly growing area and previously little focus has been placed on it. With the continued increase in funding within professional sport, this area is now coming to the fore, with ongoing continued research being carried out.

However, there are increased high-level evidence papers in the sports medical literature to support the previously anecdotal evidence of poor dental health in sportspeople and also demonstrating the benefits and championing the cause for routine dental screening. Several positions and consensus statements with recommendations to promote oral health screening and related research, as part of sport and exercise medicine have also been published [59,61].

Many sporting bodies are now advocating dental screens and dental fitness to compete prior to seasons starting or embarking on overseas tours and major competitions. However, few teams integrate oral health promotion within overall medical care, and there is, at present, a lack of ongoing support and reinforcement of this health area for the athletes.

In conjunction with oral health screening, the recognition and immediate care of dental traumatic injuries is critical to the athlete continuation of play and participation. Once the player is managed initially then they will require definitive ongoing restorative care.

Being a team dentist or sports dentist can be very rewarding and satisfying. It allows professional sporting relationships to be formed with team staff and players. This can give a pleasant diversion from the hustle and bustle of day-to-day general practice. It also gives the dental healthcare professional the chance to be part of something special with your own local team or sports club.

Improved oral health will positively impact athlete quality of life, wellbeing, and psychological preparedness for sport. The existing data also supports oral health education of youth football players, given the increase in oral disease with age and this should be adopted across other age grade sports.

Efficient and effective dental screening has the potential to reduce oral health inequalities. Estai et al. [62] discuss in their literature future screening tools for remote dental screening, which are gaining popularity in research. This is the use of a 'tele health system' whereby photographs of the patients' dentition are taken and emailed to the dental practitioner for assessment. This is currently in use in under-served populations in remote Alaska and Australia [63]. This is something that potentially could be expanded on or trialed within sport if difficulties in access to the dental surgery are a problem, as previously outlined with overseas training bases or competitions. As dental professionals, we must also strive to continue to collate high-quality data to add to the growing bank of data to further strengthen and change attitudes regarding dental health screening.

Therefore there is a need to shift dental sporting culture from a quick cure to a care culture, being proactive rather than reactive regarding dental health.

References

1 Studen-Pavlovich, D., Bonci, L., Etzel, K.R. (2000). Dental implications of nutritional factors in young athletes. *Dental Clinics of North America* 44(1): 161–178.

2 Chander, S., Rees, J.S. (2010). Strategies for the prevention of erosive tooth surface loss. *Dental Update* 37(1): 12–4.

3 Pennock, A., Russell, M. (2011). Dietary analysis of young professional soccer players for 1 week during the competitive season. *Journal of Strength and Conditioning Research* 25(7): 1816–1823.

4 Rees, J.S. (2004). The role of drinks in tooth surface loss. *Dental Update* 31(6): 318–320, 322–324, 326.

5 Sirimaharaj, V., Brearley Messer, L., Morgan, M.V. (2002). Acidic diet and dental erosion among athletes. *Australian Dental Journal* 47(3): 228–236.

6 Noble, W.H., Donovan, T.E., Geissberger, M. (2011). Sports drinks and dental erosion. *Journal of Californian Dental Association* 39(4): 233–238.

7 Buczkowska-Radlinska, J., Lagocka, R., Kaczmarek, W., Gorski, M., Nowicka, A. (2012). Prevalence of dental erosion in adolescent competitive swimmers exposed to gas chlorinated swimming pool water. *Clinical Oral Investigation* 17(2): 579–583.

8 Dawes, C., Boroditsky, C. (2008). Rapid and severe tooth erosion from swimming in an improper chlorinated pool: case report. *Journal of Canadian Dental Association* 74 (4): 359–361.

9 D'Ercole, S., Martinelli, D., Tripodi, D. (2016). The effect of swimming on oral health status: competitive versus non competitive athletes. *Journal of Applied Oral Science* 24 (2): 107–113.

10 Zebrauskas, A., Birskute, R., Maciulskiene, V. (2014). Prevalence of dental erosion among the young regular swimmers in Kaunas, Lithuania. *Journal of Oral Maxillofacial Research* 5(2): 1–7.

11 Geurtsen, W. (2000). Rapid general dental erosion by gas-chlorinated swimming pool water. Review of the literature and case report. *American Journal of Dentistry* 13(6): 291–293.

12 Milosevic, A., Kelly, M., McLean, A. (1997). Sports supplement drinks and dental health in competitive swimmers and cyclists. *British Dental Journal.* 182(8): 303–308.

13 Ranalli, D.N. (2002). Sports dentistry and dental traumatology. *Dental Traumatology* 18: 231–236.

14 Persson, L.G., Kiliaridis, S. (1994). Dental injuries, temporomandibular disorders, and caries in wrestlers. *Scandanavian Journal of Dental Research* 102(6): 367–371.

15 Sankaranarayanan, R. (2014). Screening for cancer in low and middle income countries. *Annals of Global Health* 80: 412–417.

16 Shiller, W. (1965). Aerodontalgia under hyperbaric conditions. *Oral Surgery, Oral Medicine and Oral Pathology* 20(5): 694–697.

17 Ashley, P., Cole, E., Diorio, A., Tanday, A., Needleman, I. (2014). Elite athletes and oral health: a review. *British Journal of Sports Medicine* 48(7): 561–562.

18 Bryant, S., McLaughlin, K., Morgaine, K., Drummond, B. (2011). Elite athletes and oral health. *International Journal Sports Medicine* 32(9): 720–724.

19 Callaghan, M.J., Jarvis, C. (1996). Evaluation of elite British cyclists: the role of the squad medical. *British Journal Sports Medicine* 30(4): 349–353.

20 De Sant'Anna, G.R., Simionato, M.R., Suzuki, M.E. (2004). Sports dentistry: buccal and salivary profile of a female soccer team. *Quintessence International* 35(8): 649–652.

21 Foster, M. (2000). Sports dentistry: what's it all about? *Journal of the South African Dental Association* 64(5): 198, 200–202, 204.

22 Inouye, J., McGrew, C. (2015). Dental problems in athletes. *Curriculum Sports Medicine* 14(1): 27–33.

23 Ljungberg, G., Birkhed, D. (1990). Dental caries in players belonging to a Swedish soccer team. *Swedish Dental Journal* 14(6): 261–266.

24 Meehan, L., Collard, M. (2013). Sports dentistry. Part 2: Dental trauma and mouth guards. *Journal of the British Society of Dental Hygiene and Therapy* 52(5): 15–22.

25 Mehrotra, V., Sawhny, A., Garg, K., Gaur, S., Hussain, J. (2014). Pain in a plane: a case report and review on barodontalgia. *International Journal of Advanced Biotechnology and Research* 5(2): 214–218.

26 McGovern, L.A., Spolarich, A.E., Keim, R. (2015). A survey of attitudes, behaviors, and needs of team dentists. *General Dentistry* 63(6): 61–66.

27 Reid, B.C., Chenette, R., Macek, M.D. (2003). Special Olympics: the oral health status of U.S. athletes compared with international athletes. *Special Care Dentist* 23(6): 230–233.

28 Soler Badia, D., Batchelor, P.A., Sheiham, A. (1994). The prevalence of oral health problems in participants of the 1992

Olympic Games in Barcelona. *International Dental Journal* 44(1): 44–48.

29 Vougiouklakis, G., Tzoutzas, J., Farmakis, E.T., et al. (2008). Dental data of the Athens 2004 Olympic and Paralympic Games. *International Journal of Sports Medicine* 29(11): 927–933.

30 Barbour, M.E., Rees, G.D. (2006). The role of erosion, abrasion, and attrition in tooth wear. *Journal Clinical Dentistry* 17(4): 88–93.

31 Gay-Escoda, C., Vieira-Duarte-Pereira, D.M., Ardèvol, J. et al. Study of the effect of oral health on physical condition of professional soccer players of the Football Club Barcelona. *Medicina oral, patología oral y cirugía bucal* 16(3): e436–e439.

32 Dellavia, C., Allievi, C,. Pallavera, A., Rosati, R., Sforza, C. (2009). Oral health conditions in Italian special Olympic athletes. *Special Care Dentist* 29(2): 69–74.

33 Fernandez, J.B., Lim, L.J., Dougherty, N., et al. (2012). Oral health findings in athletes with intellectual disabilities at the NYC Special Olympics. *Special Care Dentist* 32(5): 205–209.

34 Leroy, R., Declerck, D., Marks, L. (2012).The oral health status of Special Olympics athletes in Belgium. *Community Dental Health* 29(1): 68–73.

35 Newsome, P., Owen, S., Reaney, D. (2010). The dentist's role in prevention of sports related oro facial injuries. *International Dentistry South Africa* 12: 50–58.

36 Ranalli, D.N. (2000). *Advances in Sports Dentistry*. W.B. Saunders Co., Philadelphia.

37 White, J.A., Beltrán, E.D., Malvitz, D.M., Perlman, S.P. (1998). Oral health status of special athletes in the San Francisco Bay Area. *Journal Californian Dental Association* 26(5): 347–354.

38 Jiang Yang, X., Schamach, P., Ping Dai, J., et al. (2011). Dental service in 2008 Summer Olympic Games. *British Journal of Sports Medicine* 45: 270–274.

39 Needleman, I., Ashley, P., Petrie, A., et al. (2013). Oral health and impact on performance of athletes participating in the London 2012 Olympic Games: a cross-sectional study. *British Journal of Sports Medicine* 47(16): 1054–1058.

40 Piccininni, P., Fasel, R. (2004). Sports dentistry and the Olympic Games. *Californian Dental Journal* 33(6): 471–483.

41 Needleman, I., Ashley, P., Meehan, L., et al. (2016). Poor oral health including active caries in 187 UK professional male football players: clinical dental examination performed by dentists. *British Journal of Sports Medicine* 50(1): 41–44.

42 Foster, M., Readman, P. (2009). Sports dentistry: what's it all about? *Dental Update* 36(3): 135–141.

43 Kini, P., Jathanna, V., Jathanna, R., Shetty, K. (2015). Barodontalgia: etiology, features and Prevention. *Open Journal of Dentistry and Oral Medicine* 3(2): 35–38.

44 Winters, J.E. (1996). Sports dentistry: the profession's role in athletics. *Journal of American Dental Association* 127: 810–811.

45 Zadik, Y. (2009). Barodontalgia. *Journal of Endodontics* 35(4): 481–485.

46 Robichaud, R., McNally, M. (2005). Barodontalgia as a differential diagnosis: symptoms and findings. *Journal of Canadian Dental Association* 71(1): 39–42.

47 Jagger, R., Jackson, S., Jagger, D. (1997). In at the deep end: an insight into scuba diving and related dental problem for the GDP. *British Dental Journal* 183(10): 380–382.

48 Health and Safety Executive. (2015). The Medical Examination and Assessment of Commercial Divers (MA1). www.hse.gov.uk/diving/amedsapproval.htm (accessed April 2018).

49 Llewellyn, C.D., Johnson, N.W., Warnakulasuriya, K.A. (2001). Risk factors for squamous cell carcinoma of the oral cavity in young people--a comprehensive literature review. *Oral Oncology* 37(5): 401–418.

50 Epstein, J.,Villines, D., Drahos, G., Kaufman, E., Gorsky, M. (2008). Oral lesions in patients participating in an oral examination screening week at an urban dental school. *Journal American Dental Association* 139(10): 1338–1344.

51 Sciubba, J.J. (1999). Improving detection of precancerous and cancerous oral lesions. Computer-assisted analysis of the oral brush biopsy. *Journal of the American Dental Association* 130(10): 1445–1457.

52 Kumamoto, D., Winters, J. (2000). Private practice and community activities in Sports Dentistry Advances in sports dentistry. *Dental Clinics of North America* 44(1): 209–220.

53 Richardson, P. (2005). Dental morbidity in United Kingdom Armed Forces Iraq 2003. *Military Medicine* 170(6): 536–541.

54 Richardson, P. (2005). Dental risk assessment for military personnel. *Military Medicine* (170)6: 542–545.

55 Needleman, I., Ashley, P., Weiler, R., McNally, S. (2016). Oral health screening should be routine in professional football: a call to action for sports and exercise medicine (SEM) clinicians. *British Journal of Sports Medicine* 50: 1289.

56 Kidd, E. (2010). Caries control from cradle to grave. *Dental Update* 37(10): 651–652, 654–656.

57 Lawson, S. (2010). Practical suggestions for implementing caries control and recall protocols for children and young adults. *Dental Update* 37(10): 709.

58 Greenberg, B., Kantor, M., Jiang, S., Glick, M. (2012). Patients attitudes toward screening for medical conditions in a dental setting. *Journal of Public Health Dentistry* 72: 28–35.

59 World Dental Federation (2017). FDI Policy statement on Sports Dentistry. *International Dental Journal* 67: 18–19.

60 Glassman, P., Anderson, M., Jacobsen, P. (2003). Practical protocols for the prevention of dental disease in community settings for people with special needs: the protocols. *Special Care Dentist* 23(5): 160–164.

61 Needleman, I., Ashley, P., Fine, P., et al. (2014). Consensus statement: oral health and elite sport performance. *British Dental Journal* 217(10): 587–590.

62 Estai, M., Winters, J., Kanagasingham, Y., et al. (2016). Validity and reliability of remote dental screening by different oral health professional using a store and forward telehealth model. *British Dental Journal* 221(7): 411–414.

63 Page, J., Kidd, E. (2010). Practical suggestions for implementing caries control and recall protocols for children and young adults. *Dental Update* 37: 422–432.

11

Delivering Dental Facilities at Sporting Events

John Haughey

11.1 Introduction

There are many challenges to providing dental support to athletes, both during training and in competition. Some of these will differ, depending on whether the athlete competes individually or as part of a team, or whether the sports dentistry support is as an ongoing relationship or at a one-off competition, and if it is a one-off, whether the competition is a single event, multiple events, or part of a multi-sport event.

In this chapter, we will discuss how a dentist can provide dental support for athletes in these different scenarios. We will consider the challenges in providing a comprehensive service at major sporting events, as well as more manageable small, local sports days.

A common challenge in all these scenarios is gaining access to the athlete to start the relationship. Even though in recent years the awareness of the importance of sports dentistry is improving across the sporting world, there is still a lack of perceived value by most athletes, coaches, and team managers. This is a major challenge for a dentist looking to get involved with sports dentistry and to help support athletes. It is less of a challenge at the elite end of some sports and sporting events, where dental support is already operating and respected, for example, NFL American football teams, NBA basketball teams, the Olympic Games and Premier League football

in the UK. The major challenge is when a dentist is looking to get involved with local athletes and teams, especially if the team or athletes are at an elite level and have not already embraced the importance of sports dentistry support. The dentist will need be to be proactive in promoting their service by showing the sport and/or athlete what the dentist has to offer, not only in dealing with immediate trauma, but with long-term advice about oral health, prevention of disease and trauma, and how dentistry is a part of general health.

When deciding on providing dental support for an athlete, whether as an individual or a team, a dentist must acknowledge that currently sports dentistry is not necessarily profitable and in most cases, it is economically negative. Accepting this and choosing athletes that are involved in a sport with which the dentist has an interest or passion will provide the most reward for the dentist.

When providing sports dentistry support to an athlete or team it is important to understand that you will be part of a much wider medical support team. With some athletes or teams you will support independently of the medical team, although the most effective support is provided when working as part of the medical team. In supporting teams there is usually at least one medical professional already in place providing support. Most commonly it is a physiotherapist. Getting to

Sports Dentistry: Principles and Practice, First Edition. Edited by Peter D. Fine, Chris Louca and Albert Leung.
© 2019 John Wiley & Sons Ltd. Published 2019 by John Wiley & Sons Ltd.
Companion website: www.wiley.com/go/fine/sports_dentistry

know the medical support team and discussing how sports dentistry support is provided, and how a sports dentist can work as part of the medical team is important for creating the best environment to provide sports dentistry support. This may involve having to convince our medical colleagues of the value of having a dentist on the team, not only from the dental trauma point of view, but from a general health perspective. Some of the best ambassadors we have to help us with this are athletes themselves, who have benefitted from a dental intervention.

11.2 Types of Sports Dentistry Support

Depending on the level of sports dentistry support being provided by the dentist to the athlete, all or some of the following services may be offered:

- Dental screening
- General dental treatment support
- Preventative care
- Mouth guard provision
- Emergency care on-site to the competition (field of play)
- Emergency care off-site to the competition
- Referral pathway.

11.2.1 Dental Screening

We look at the importance and significance of dental screening of athletes in more depth in Chapter 10, but dental screening is an important part of the sports dentistry support for athletes. It allows an opportunity to set up regular contact with the athletes, allowing continued development of the relationship between the athlete and the dentist.

The dental screening of individual athletes can be done during a normal examination appointment at the supporting dental practice. When supporting a team it is very impractical and in most cases impossible to get all members of a team to the dental practice in a reasonable time frame to carry out the dental examinations. Mobile dental screenings are particularly relevant when working with teams as it allows an effective way to provide support to a high number of athletes in a time-efficient manner (Figure 11.1).

Athletes and teams generally break up their year into three seasons, pre-season, in-season, and off-season. Establishing a regular allocation for the dental screening to take place is important to ensure it is not overlooked and continues on an annual basis. The recommended time to carry out the dental screening is in the pre-season. In pre-season a

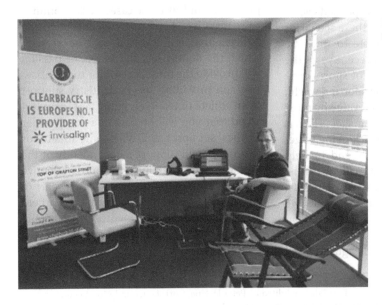

Figure 11.1 An example of an on-site screening facility.

lot of physical and medical screenings of the athletes and fitness tests take place to provide baselines and planning for the season ahead. This makes pre-season a natural fit for the dental screening to take place. An annual dental screening will allow the athlete to get a dental health clearance for the year ahead. For athletes taking part in contact sports, this is also a good opportunity to provide a custom-fitted mouth guard for the season ahead.

11.2.2 General Dental Treatment Support

A recent systemic review [1] on the oral health of elite athletes stated oral health of athletes is poor, therefore there is a high chance when a dentist starts to provide support to an athlete they may need some general dental treatment to become dentally healthy. Some important considerations that a dentist should understand before they offer general dental treatment to athletes include cost, time, and perceived value.

11.2.2.1 Cost
The cost of the treatment is an important consideration that will need to be discussed in advance with the athlete. Most full-time amateur athletes, including some Olympians, have limited funding and need to prioritise their spending. It may be difficult for the athlete to see the value in paying for dental treatment when they are under financial pressure with training, competing, travelling, medical support, and living costs. Professional athletes may also have financial pressures, especially if they are not achieving at the high end of their sport.

The dentist needs to establish a clear understanding with the athlete about the cost of the treatment. Options include full dental practice prices, reduced prices, or as pro bono. Dental treatment carried out at a reduced price or as pro bono can be balanced out by forming an agreement with the athlete that they will use their profile to market the practice through social media, media, and

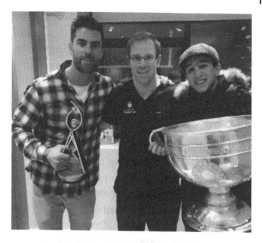

Figure 11.2 Practice building via social media.

word of mouth. This can be very successful as a practice builder (Figure 11.2).

11.2.2.2 Time
To carry out the dental treatment on athletes will need time, firstly from the athlete to attend the dental practice and secondly out of the dentist's appointment book.

Full-time amateur and professional athletes, unless in acute dental pain, are unlikely take time away from their normal training routine to attend the dental practice. Before offering to provide dental treatment support, the dentist needs to consider the times and days that the athlete will attend the dental practice and ensure that they can facilitate dental appointments at these times. Alternatively, the dentist will need to consider what time he/she can offer their services to the sports team or individual athlete and attend their sports arena.

The amount of surgery time at the dental practice allocated to providing general dental treatment to athletes needs to be considered before the dentist commits themselves to providing comprehensive dental treatment. If the dental treatment is being paid for by the athlete at normal practice prices then it is less of a consideration. If it is at a reduced price or as pro bono then this will have an impact on the practice turnover. It may be minimal if the dentist chooses to only support a selected number of athletes. Where the dentist is supporting a team/club this could have a major impact on practice turnover. This may be a potential barrier to providing this support, especially if the dentist providing the support is not the owner of the practice or is a single-handed practitioner.

11.2.2.3 Perceived Value

The perceived value of the dental treatment to the athlete will impact on the dentist's cost and time to provide the treatment.

Like any patient, if the athlete values their dental health and the treatment needed to ensure it is optimised, then they will always be on time for their appointments and will gladly pay full cost for expensive dental treatment. In reality, their dental health is not high on their list of priorities and many other commitments may cause the athlete to change their appointment at late notice or not attend with no notice given. As sports dentists, we have to appreciate that elite athletes are generally only interested in what will improve their performance and not how having their teeth checked regularly may influence their health. They are not interested in health – only performance – and so taking time to go to the dentist when they don't have a dental problem will be seen as time that could be better spent training, resting, or eating. A dentist should take this into consideration, and understand the challenge of encouraging an athlete to value their oral health.

If a dentist is providing dental treatment for athletes at a reduced price or as pro bono then a simple way to successfully provide general dental treatment for athletes is to allocate one to two hours per month for athletes. These hours could be outside the normal scheduled surgery hours for the dentist, therefore having no negative impact on turnover. The one to two hours should be at a time and day of the week that is accessible for the athletes. This will allow a platform for a dentist to provide general dental treatment support to athletes without the possible frustrations of cost, time, and perceived value

affecting the dentist's experience and straining the relationship with the athlete or team. For example, if a local sports team give their elite athletes an afternoon away from training on a certain day then that would be a good time to offer availability to surgery time.

11.2.3 Preventative Care

A preventative care programme can be provided independently or in combination with the dental screening and general dental treatment. Similar to the general patient, this should include regular examination, radiographs, and hygiene treatment. This will also provide an opportunity to reinforce good oral health habits and to continue to build a positive relationship with the athlete.

For the individual athlete, an annual dental appointment, including a full dental examination, scale and polish, any necessary radiographs, reinforcement of the importance of good oral health, and provision of a custom-fitted mouth guard, if needed, would be an effective preventive programme.

For a team, an annual off-site screening, including a custom-fitted mouth guard service, followed by a visit to the practice for reinforcement of good oral hygiene techniques, scale and polish, and any necessary radiographs would be ideal.

11.2.3.1 Mouth Guard Provision

A custom-fitted, pressurised, thermoformed, laminated mouth guard is recommended in contact sports to reduce the risk of traumatic dental injuries. This is another service a dentist can provide to athletes.

We look at the importance of mouth guards as a preventative measure in Chapter 7. There is a lack of knowledge and value from athletes and coaches on the different types of mouth guards and which one is recommended. An example of the lack of value placed on the correct type of mouth guard was demonstrated in a small study (J Haughey, unpublished) carried out at the Commonwealth Games in Glasgow 2014.

Of the 104 boxers who competed at the quarter-final stage, 49% were wearing boil-and-bite mouth guards. These were athletes competing for their country at the latter stages of an international tournament in a sport where it is compulsory to wear a mouth guard. For over a week a free custom-fitted mouth guard service was available at the Athletes' Village where the athletes were staying. Access, time, and cost was no barrier to getting a custom-fitted mouth guard in this scenario, and still so many athletes continued to wear a boil-and-bite mouth guard. One of these athletes lacerated the lingual surface of their upper lip during their next competition. The laceration occurred adjacent to a rough surface edge on their mouth guard (Figures 11.3–11.6).

Providing mouth guard provision for athletes is easily implemented. The service can be provided in the dental practice or at an on-site visit. In providing an on-site mouth guard service it is important to have organised an effective process and ensure adequate materials are available on-site. The service can be done as part of a screening visit or as independent mouth guard provision visits.

A sample mouth guard fitting protocol for a team is as follows.

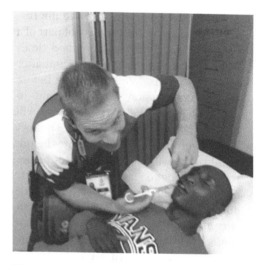

Figure 11.5 Treatment of injury.

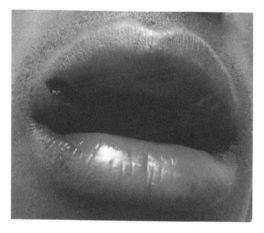

Figure 11.3 Oral laceration suffered during competition.

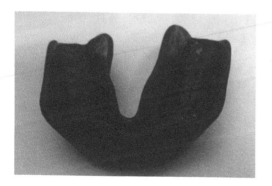

Figure 11.4 Mouth guard worn at time of injury.

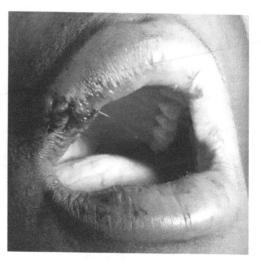

Figure 11.6 Treated soft tissue injury with sutures.

On-site mouth guard protocol:

1) *Pre-impression screening.* If a prior dental screening has not been done and this is the first time you will see the athlete, it is important to establish that they are dentally fit for an alginate impression. A medical/dental questionnaire and consent form can be created and sent to the athlete prior to the visit to confirm that they are dentally fit for a mouth guard impression. A small screen can also be carried out at the visit, if time allows.

2) *Organize visit.* Discuss with your team point of contact to organize the impression visit. If the impression is not part of a planned screening visit then good times to make impressions are before and after training sessions. When planning before the training session it is important to allow adequate time so that the visit will not interfere with training plans. The visit could involve setting up 60 minutes before training and will finish 10 minutes before training is due to start, to ensure there is no negative effect on player attendance during training. When the date of the visit is confirmed, advise your team point of contact to inform the athletes that anyone wanting a mouth guard needs to turn up early for training to receive an impression.

After visit dates are confirmed, enquire about the facilities present at the ground. Organize to have access to the first aid room or another suitable room, and confirm if the team medical staff will be present in case of a medical emergency during the visit.

3) *Visit setup.* When setting up at the visit, make sure to take into consideration appropriate cross-infection procedures. This should include a clean environment, zoning with designated clean and dirty zones and appropriate disinfection (Figure 11.7). Make sure there is adequate lighting if you plan to do a quick dental screening.

4) *Visit protocol.* Players should be organized to attend for an impression by the team point of contact or an allocated responsible person to ensure the most efficient use of the time. When a player arrives, they can fill in the medical/dental questionnaire and sign the consent form to have an upper alginate impression made if they haven't prior to the visit. When they are seated in the impression chair, perform a quick dental screening. If you feel they are medically and dentally fit for an alginate impression, proceed in making the impression. The impression

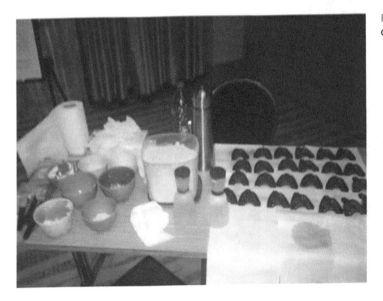

Figure 11.7 An example of on-site impression facilities.

should be disinfected and bagged immediately after it is removed from the mouth in an air-tight sealed bag, and a laboratory form should be filled out and placed in the bag pocket. If the dental screening identified any dental needs, the player should be given an advice summary form.

5) *Sending to lab.* The impressions should be appropriately boxed and sent to your chosen laboratory for the fabrication of pressurised thermoformed laminated mouthgaurds.

6) *Fitting of mouth guards.* A dentist is required to fit the mouth guards when they are received back from the laboratory. The mouth guards from an earlier impression visit can be linked in with any further impression visits, if planned, to allow adequate turnaround time from the laboratory. Otherwise, discuss with the team point of contact to organise a suitable fit visit for the mouth guards.

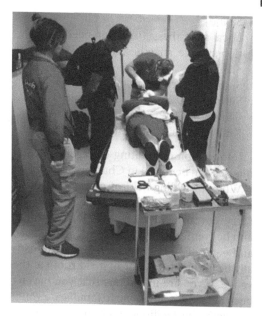

Figure 11.8 Providing support during Rio Olympic Games 2016.

11.2.4 Emergency Care On-site

When providing on-site or field-of-play emergency dental care you will be part of the medical support team (Figure 11.8). Depending on the level of support the team or athlete has, this could include some or all of the following: physiotherapists, sports medicine doctor, massage therapist, nutritionist, performance psychologist, and sports nurse.

It is important to see yourself as part of this team and familiarise yourself with everyone's roles. As part of the support team, and depending on the depth of support, you may be of benefit to the team or athlete using your non-conventional dental skills. For example, you may assist in the removal of an athlete from the field of play in a medical emergency or injury scenario. Using your suturing skills to help provide wound closure of superficial skin lacerations is another valuable contribution. These extra skills will provide more depth in your support to the athlete or team and will help in the acceptance of dental support being onsite.

As a general rule and to ensure you are supported by your medical defence society, you should not provide treatment that you have not been trained to do or that you do not feel confident and competent in doing.

As a field-of-play dentist, it is important to have an adequate dental kit to provide first-stage treatment in any dental emergency. It is important that you stock the field-of-play kit and are responsible for it being present during your field-of-play support. An example of such a kit is given below.

Field-of-play dental kit:

- Headlight (runner's headlights are good here)
- Examination kits (mirror, probe, tweezers)
- Ward's carver
- Gauze
- Cotton rolls
- Flowable composite
- Composite resin
- Cordless light curing lamp
- Splinting material (orthodontic wire, titanium trauma splint)
- Etch
- Bond
- Desensitizer

- Saline
- Local anaesthesia (injection needles, injection syringe, anaethesic)
- Sharps box
- Suture kit (artery forceps, scissors)
- Sutures (4/0 and 5/0 Vircyl Rapide)
- Gloves
- Kit bag to carry your kit.

Information on treating emergency dental injuries can be found in Chapters 2, 3 and 4.

When providing field-of-play support it is important to understand where you will carry out any emergency dental treatment and be comfortable you have adequate space and equipment (Figure 11.9). This will usually be in the medical or first aid room at the venue. If you are in a venue that you haven't been before it is advisable to familiarise yourself with the facilities, and speak with the other medical personnel so there is a clear understanding of what the procedure is in the event of a dental emergency.

11.2.5 Emergency Care Off-site

Off-site emergency care support can be provided to sports teams and athletes independently or in conjunction with

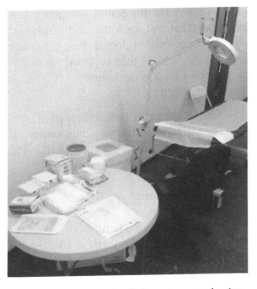

Figure 11.9 An example of adequate space, boxing event at Baku Islamic Solidarity Games, 2017.

field-of-play emergency care. Before offering this service to a sports team or athlete, the dentist must be comfortable with being able to access dental clinic facilities during the times that most sports are played, which is usually in the evenings or at weekends.

If it is an independent service, as in there is no field-of-play support, then a protocol needs to be put in place with the head of medical support for the team, which is usually the head physiotherapist. The medical lead or other appropriately designated individual should be trained by the dentist on how to react to a dental emergency and then initiate the process so the athlete can be seen in the dental clinic as soon as possible.

The dental clinic that will facilitate the emergency treatment should be within an appropriate travel time from the competition venue; allowing the treatment to be administrated within a time period that will provide the most favourable outcome for the treatment. A process should be in place for the dentist to be contactable, if they are not on-site when an incident happens, and for transport of the athlete from the venue to the dental clinic.

Setting up a network of dentists to provide emergency care off-site at each of the venues the athlete or team competes at would be a more robust option. If the athlete or team regularly compete at venues that are not within an appropriate travel time to the clinic then the treatment outcome of a dental emergency may suffer if support local to the competition venue is not provided; for example, if a dentist providing support to a team that plays against other teams in a home and away fixture league, where the away fixtures travel time following a dental emergency is greater than 4 hours. In this scenario, working with the dentists supporting the other teams in the league will create a network of dental clinics local to each competition venue providing emergency dental care. This will allow the most favourable treatment outcomes for any athlete at any venue in that league.

11.3   Referral Pathway

A referral pathway for dental emergencies outside the scope of practice of the supporting dentist needs to be considered, for example, following mandibular and maxillary fractures.

The referral pathway can include a range of support from using the nearest accident and emergency department to having a specific maxillo-facial or plastic surgeon as part of the off-site medical support. This will depend on a number of things, including cost and who is covering the cost. If the dentist is not providing field-of-play support, then the process they have in place needs to be understood by the medical lead on the day of competition.

11.4   Sports Dentistry Support for the Individual Athlete

Supporting the individual athlete has a different dynamic to supporting a team and may allow more in-depth dental support due to less demand on surgery time. Individual athletes have smaller support teams around them due to the athlete in most cases having to cover the financial costs themselves. Contact with the individual athlete is generally done directly or in some cases through their manager.

Some or all of the following support can be provided to the individual athlete.

11.4.1   Dental Screening

Ideally, an annual dental screening carried out in the dental surgery should be provided. Depending on the training and competition schedule and the location of the athlete, a regular annual slot in the practice during pre-season can be scheduled. It is important to realise that compared to a normal patient, the individual athlete may need a more intensive reminder system due to their irregular training and competition schedule and the value they place on sports dentistry support.

11.4.2   General Dental Treatment Support

Any treatment needed to help develop and maintain optimum oral health for the athlete can be provided in the dental clinic.

- *Preventative care.* A regular hygiene programme can be set up through the hygiene services in the clinic. The frequency may be dependent on the availability of the athlete.
- *Mouth guard provision.* A custom-fitted pressurized thermoformed mouth guard can be provided if needed at the annual dental screening.
- *Emergency care on-site to the competition.* Field-of-play dental support could be an option in some high-risk facial and jaw injury sports. Usually it is not necessary for the individual athlete, as many of their competitions involve travelling and the cost would not be justified unless the dentist is travelling as a fan.
- *Emergency care off-site to the competition.* Adequate emergency service can be provided by the dentist making themselves contactable during competition and having access to the dental clinic.
- *Referral pathway.* A referral pathway should be set up so the dentist can provide the athlete the most efficient way to get treatment beyond the skills of the dentist, for example suspected facial and jaw fractures and facial soft tissue injuries.

11.5   Sports Dentistry Support for a Team

Supporting a team has different challenges to supporting the individual athlete. The first challenge will be to get the offer to provide support accepted. Unless it is a professional team that already understands the importance of sport dentistry, the dentist will need to be proactive and provide justification to the decision-makers for them to introduce this new support to their athletes.

The time needed to provide an adequate support service and the logistics of organising a group of people will be the biggest challenge.

The point of contact will differ depending on the size of support the team has. A local small sports club usually will have only one manager who is responsible for organising everything from the team. In this case they will be the point of contact. A larger team will have a management team and possibly a dedicated physiotherapist who attends their competitions and training. In this case one of the management team or the physiotherapist depending on the service provided may be the point of contact.

Some or all of the following support can be provided to the team:

- *Dental screening.* The annual dental screen will be most efficiently done at the training ground of the team. It is unlikely all the members of the team will attend the dental clinic in adequate time to complete the screening. This is best done during the pre-season and it is logistically easier to include it as part of the medical screening that is generally already in place. If regular medical screening is not currently taking place, which will probably be the case for the local small team, then it can be carried out around training. An option could be to screen five athletes before each training session until all athletes have been screened.

- *General dental treatment support.* Any treatment indicated from the screening can be relayed back to the athlete and can be provided in the dental clinic. When booking visits to the clinic, the priority should be given to the athletes with the greatest need identified at the screening. It will be important to explain the consequences to performance of not getting treatment to both the athlete and the management. This will prevent a scenario where an athlete does not attend for treatment after being advised of the need from the screening. It should be emphasised that having identified treatment required at the screening, which may need to be undertaken as a matter of urgency, the athlete is free to seek that treatment from whichever dental practitioner they wish. The relative urgency of treatment should be explained to the athlete, the medical team, and the management team, so that dental emergencies may be avoided during the season, when missing a training session or match may be most inconvenient.

- *Preventative care.* A regular hygiene programme can be set up through the hygiene services in the clinic for all athletes. The frequency may be dependent on the availability of the athletes.

- *Mouth guard provision.* A new custom-fitted pressurized thermoformed mouth guard can be provided at the annual dental screening. The impression can be taken after the screen and a second date can be organised for the fitting.

- *Emergency care on-site to the competition.* Field-of-play dental support could be an option in some high-risk facial and jaw injury sports. In this situation the dentist will work as part of the medical team where the physiotherapist is usually the head of the medical support and will be lead medic during the competition. A dentist supporting the medical team of a major sporting team, for example a Premier League football team in England and Wales, may well travel with the team, but more usually the medical support of the home team would cover both sides in the event of serious orofacial/dental injuries.

- *Emergency care off-site to the competition.* Adequate emergency services can be provided by the dentist having access to the dental clinic during competition. If the dentist is also giving field-of-play support they can transfer the athlete to the practice for treatment. If the dentist is not giving field-of-play support then a process where the dentist can be contacted by the lead medic on the day and the athlete transported from the competition to the dental practice will need to be in place.

- *Referral pathway.* A referral pathway should be set up so the dentist can provide the athlete with the most efficient way to get treatment beyond the skills of the dentist, for example suspected facial and jaw fractures and facial soft tissue injuries.

11.6 Sports Dentistry Support at a Competition

The role of the sports dentist at a local competition differs from dental support of an individual athlete or a team, as the dentist will support all the athletes. There is no reason for individual athletes to have their own personal dental support, provided the dental support at the competition is well trained in the needs of athletes.

Some or all of the following support can be provided at a competition:

- *Dental screening.* A dental screening of the athletes taking part in the competition may be too difficult to co-ordinate, especially in a competition were athletes arrive and leave on the day of competition.
- *Emergency care on-site for the competition.* Field-of-play dental support as part of the athlete medical team can be provided. It is important to get to know the medical team before the day of competition so everyone's role is clear and understood.
- *Emergency care off-site for the competition.* Access to the dental clinic during competition and transport for athletes from the competition to the dental practice will need to be in place. An important consideration here is that if the dentist needs to have a colleague on call, to provide cover in the event that the competition is still in progress and an athlete needs to attend the dental clinic for treatment.
- *Referral pathway.* A referral pathway should be set up so the dentist can provide

the athlete with the most efficient way to get treatment for suspected facial and jaw fractures.

11.7 Sports Dentistry Support at Major Events

The size of the tournament determines the level of sports dentistry support at a major event. For example, the London Olympics 2012 provided both general dentistry support and emergency dentistry support to the athletes and their support teams through field-of-play dentists and an on-site dental clinic. The Glasgow Commonwealth Games 2014 provided only emergency dental support to the athletes through field-of-play dentists and an on-site dental clinic, while the Islamic Solidarity Games Baku 2017 provided limited emergency dental support through a field-of-play dentist. The organising committee for the event, together with the medical team will determine the level of dental support.

The level of support will generally be determined by the amount of available funding for sports dentistry. The funding available to the organising committee will usually depend on the prestige of the event and the support of the local government. The more prestigious the event, the more interest there will be from sponsors, media broadcasters, and commercial partners, which will filter down to the available funding of the medical organising committee for the games. Dental support at major sporting events is usually free to the athletes and in the case of an Olympic Games free to the whole Olympic family.

The Olympics is the most prestigious multi-sport event in the world and therefore it provides the most comprehensive sports dentistry support of all major tournaments.

The IOC Medical Commission states, 'Since the 1920s, the IOC has supported a dental clinic for athletes and Olympic family members at every Olympic Games. At some Games, over 1000 athletes and other individuals benefited from this programme. The Olympic Dental Service has provided both emergency and required dental care, as well as a mouth guard programme for athletes participating in contact sports. As a testament to the importance of the Sports Dentistry programme at the Olympic Games, a dentist has been a member of the Medical Commission Games Group since 1999.' (https://hub.olympic.org/wp-content/uploads/2016/06/FINAL-Olympic-Dental-Brochure.pdf)

At the last Olympics, Rio 2016, the Olympic Dental Programme (https://hub.olympic.org/rio-2016/rio-olympic-dental-programme/) included:

- *Dental facilities.* An eight-chair dental clinic within the Olympic Village Polyclinic. The facility was available for one month from the start of the athletes and teams arriving at the Olympic Village until they left. Opening hours during Olympic competition was 24/7; a dentist was on-call for the duration of this period.
- *Dental services.* Emergency care was available for all members of the Olympic family, with general dental treatment restricted to athletes only and specialist dental treatment (endodontics and surgical extractions) available just for athletes.
- *Mouth guard programme.* Athletes could avail themselves of the mouth guard programme. This involved providing a custom-fitted pressurized thermoforming mouth guard with a two-day turnaround time from impression to fitting.
- *Dental screening.* The dental screening involved a dental checkup and screening radiography. A copy of the report was then provided to the athlete to take home. Athletes were encouraged to attend by the offering of a gift from the IOC for anyone who attended for a screening.
- *Dental survey.* A short (10 questions) online dental survey was also available through the athlete online platform, Athlete Hub. Participation was again encouraged through provision of a prize to anyone who completed it.

- *Venue dental coverage.* A dentist was part of the athlete medical team at the venue of sports with a higher risk of trauma to the face and mouth; these included basketball, boxing, handball, hockey, rugby, and water polo.

The medical organising committee for a major sporting event will have some important considerations when planning and developing the sports dentistry support during competition. They include:

- Level of cover
- Recruitment of dentists and dental care professionals
- Training recruits
- Types of equipment
- Legacy

11.8 Level of Cover

The level of cover will be determined by the amount of funding and the availability of facilities. Options include:

1) Partnership with local a dental practice
2) Field-of-play dentist for emergency treatment
3) On-site dental facilities for emergency and general dental treatment
4) Mouth guard programme
5) Referral service for facial and jaw fractures.

11.8.1 Partnership with a Local Dental Practice

This would be the most effective and cost-efficient support for smaller events. An agreement can be made with a local dental practice to provide emergency dental support during the competition, in return for advertising, marketing and sponsorship benefits. The organising committee will need to put in place a process that allows the dentist to be contacted and the athlete to be transported to the local dental practice in a reasonable time period from the time of the incident.

11.8.2   Field-of-play Dentist for Emergency Treatment

For sports involving a higher risk of trauma to the face and mouth, the organising committee should consider having a sports dentist as part of the athlete medical team supporting the competition. Considerations for this include the cost of equipment and remuneration for the supporting dentist. For smaller events a partnership with a local sports dentist who also has the facilities to provide follow-up treatment is preferable. For larger events where multiple venues need cover at the same time, a recruitment plan for acquiring an adequate number of sports dentists will need to be put in place by the organising committee. The planning of dental personnel and facilities needs to be considered in the context of what the organising committee considers to be reasonable facilities to offer athletes, the rationale for medical cover, the number of athletes attending, a knowledge of previous events, and funding available.

11.8.3   On-site Dental Facilities for Emergency and General Dental Treatment

On-site dental facilities are dependent on having the funding to provide the equipment, as well as having the appropriate location to set up the facility. At a major event where there will be an athlete centre, like the Athletes' Village at the Olympics, or an event where there is only one venue then this is an appropriate location for setting up an on-site dental facility. At a major event where an athlete polyclinic will be set up then the ability to also provide an on-site dental clinic will be viable. The cost of the equipment and materials, the set-up of the dental clinic, the appointment system, the recruitment of staff, the cost of treatment, and the treatments that will be offered are all challenges that need to be considered by the organising committee.

If the organising committee wants to provide simply emergency trauma cover, then facilities, equipment, and number of dental personnel will be different to if a full dental facility is required. Polyclinics, as seen at recent Olympic Games, have provided dental facilities, including six to eight fully equipped dental units, technical support, dental care professional (DCP) support, including chair-side assistance and hygienists, and reception staff.

11.8.4   Mouth Guard Programme

At an event involving sports that have a risk of facial and mouth injuries, a mouth guard could be provided. An important consideration is whether the mouth guards would be manufactured at the on-site dental facilities or by a local mouth guard manufacturer. The cost of equipment and having the appropriate staff to facilitate on-site manufacture of the mouth guards will determine which option to choose. A process will be needed for making the athlete's impression and the time it takes between impression and fitting will need to be established. If the purpose of the mouth guard programme is to provide a custom-fitted, pressurised, thermoformed mouth guard for the competition then the accessibility to athletes before the competition and the time needed to provide the mouth guard must be considered to ensure this is successful. If the mouth guard programme is to raise awareness of the importance of the correct mouth guard type and provision of such a mouth guard to the athlete to show them the benefit in preventing injury, then there is less time pressure on whether the delivery of the mouth guard programme will be a success.

Over 200 custom-fitted mouth guards were provided at London 2012, to athletes who had never had a protective mouth guard, had forgotten their mouth guard, decided they wanted a new one, or who suddenly realised the positive impact of mouth guards and therefore wanted to avail themselves of the service.

11.8.5 Referral Service for Facial and Jaw Fractures

A referral service for incidents involving possible jaw and facial fractured should be put in place, especially for sports with a higher risk. This is usually done through the local hospital.

11.9 Recruitment of Dentists and Dental Care Professionals

A major challenge to providing sports dentistry support that involves on-site dental facilities, field-of-play emergency cover, or a mouth guard programme is the recruitment of the staff who will deliver the service.

For smaller tournaments, this could be done through partnerships with local dental practices and mouth guard manufacturers. For major events a more extensive recruitment process is needed. Recruiting enough dentists and DCPs for major sporting events needs to be planned well in advance.

The sports dentists that provide cover at the Olympics are recruited through the Olympic volunteer programme under the remit of the Olympic chief dental officer, who is part of the International Olympic Committee. The Olympic chief dental officer will delegate the responsibility of providing facilities and personnel to a dental colleague, normally in the host country where the Olympics will take place. This individual will be responsible for the recruitment, training, and equipping the dental team. The dental team are part of a much larger medical team, which includes sports medicine consultants, orthopaedic surgeons, trauma specialists, sports psychologists, physiotherapists, masseurs, nutritionists, ophthalmologists, pharmacists, and all the technical support that is required. The Olympic volunteer programme involves a general application, which is followed by an interview if the application is successful and then a selection process.

Successful applicants will then be offered roles. This is the process for all Olympic volunteers, which at Rio 2016 involved 240 000 applications for the recruitment of 70 000 volunteers for the games. The process involved the use of an online platform with individual portal log in.

For smaller events, providing an online platform for recruitment and training is not financially viable. The process should involve an awareness campaign directed at sports dentists, an application process, and a selection process. The application and selection processes can be effectively achieved through email and skype by the medical organising committee for the competition. Having experience of these events can help an individual to be asked to participate in a sporting event and certainly dentists with specialist training in sports dentistry are looked upon favourably by events organisers.

11.10 Training Recruits

After staff for the sports dentistry support have been selected, a training programme is required prior to competition. The focus of the training programme should not be on the dental skills needed to provide the sports dentistry support, as the recruitment process should have selected staff that already have adequate skills. The training should be to help the staff understand about the competition, the venues, and the dental facilities at the venue where they will be working.

For example, the Olympics volunteer training programme has three areas of focus. Firstly, there is the training about the Olympics – the values, the sports, and the venues. Secondly will be the role-specific training, where dentists will take part in the medical team role-specific training. The focus is on understanding the structure and role of the medical support through the games. Lastly, the venue-specific training will take place close to the event. This will focus on the venue and sports taking place at the venue, so there is a clear understanding of the medical team roles, facilities, and processes. Knowing and understanding the customs of a host nation can help the volunteer dentist to appreciate the role that they are likely to fulfil when applying to become a volunteer. This can be important when training staff who may not be used to working odd shift patterns, hanging around between shifts, living in an Olympic-style village, working as part of a medical team, living in shared accommodation, and being away from family and routine work for an extended period of time. The initial concept of volunteering for a major sporting event or games, or even a minor sporting event, may sound attractive, but the reality is often somewhat different.

These three areas, competition-specific training, role-specific training, and venue-specific training, are a good baseline for creating a training programme for preparing the sports dentistry support staff for the competition. Depending on the size of the workforce, some of the training can be carried out online before the event.

11.11   Types of Equipment

The types of equipment needed will depend on the level of cover being provided.

Field-of-play emergency dental kits will need to be available. This is less challenging to organise, as the kit usually only includes the essentials for providing emergency dental care. The only considerations are if the organising committee or the field-of-play dentist provide the kit, what happens to the kit after the competition. An example of a field-of-play kit is detailed in Section 11.2.4.

On-site dental services provide a much greater challenge. Options vary between using mobile dental units or fixed dental units as well as the use of disposable instruments or reusable instruments. The cost of setting up an on-site dental service will determine the type of equipment used in most cases. This can be offset by looking for

options to reduce the cost. Deciding to lease the equipment or getting a dental equipment provider to loan the equipment as part of a sponsorship deal may be an option if the prestige of the event is attractive to the supplier. There are some companies who provide on-site dental services to the corporate environment and hiring the equipment from them may be a cost-effective option.

The uniform of the dental staff should also be considered. At major events there is generally a set uniform for staff that will apply to the dentists involved as well. There may be a set uniform to identify the medical team for the competition, which will apply to the dentists.

11.12   Legacy

The legacy of the sports dentistry support at a major competition like the Olympics can have a major impact. The equipment used for the on-site dental clinic with the support of the local government can be used to set up a dental clinic in a local area where the demand is greatest. Part of the legacy of the London 2012 Olympic Games was to provide a medical centre (including dentistry) for the residents of Stratford, London, which was achieved.

The survey and screening results can provide valuable information about the oral health of elite athletes from multiple sports. This can be used to help increase awareness of the importance of the athlete's oral health to the sporting community. A good example of this is the work done by Prof Ian Needleman and UCL Eastman from London 2012 (see Chapter 9).

The sports dentistry support at a smaller competition can also leave a great legacy. Whether it is emergency dental support, general dental support, or a mouth guard programme, every interaction with an athlete, coach, or sports medical practitioner is an opportunity to raise awareness of the importance of oral health in athletes.

11.13   Conclusion

Hopefully this chapter affords some understanding of the challenges when providing dental support to athletes and at sporting events. Sports dentistry support is a growing field and the importance of promoting the value of sports dentistry to athletes, coaches, and managers cannot be understated. It can be frustrating when trying to provide dental support to athletes if the same value you put on this support is not shared by the athletes and their support team. This is why one of the best pieces of advice I can give is to make sure you are providing support in a sport that you have a passion about, as the experiences will outweigh the frustrations you will face when trying to provide the best sports dentistry support possible.

I have had some fantastic experiences in my time in sports dentistry, including being a field-of-play dentist at major events, including the last two Olympic Games, providing ongoing local sports dentistry support to very successful athletes and teams, as well as launching an oral health programme for the 2000+ members of an elite players' body. One thing it has not been is financially beneficial, but the experiences and relationships that develop make it much more rewarding to this sports-mad dentist.

Recently, I have had the pleasure of reflecting on my journey in sports dentistry. I was with an athlete that I first came across five years previously, while volunteering at the London Olympics in 2012. At the Games, I barely knew his name and had no relationship with him. I witnessed him winning an Olympic medal while I was a field-of-play dentist at the venue. Two years later I was a volunteer field-of-play dentist at the Glasgow Commonwealth Games and was part of the athlete medical team that helped him with a deep laceration on his forehead suffered during his competition (Figure 11.10). He was able to pass his medical the next day and win gold in the final. Shortly after this, even though he lived a two hour drive away, he availed himself of my sports dentistry support, providing dental screening, general dental care, preventative care and mouth guard provision. The following year the national coach of his sport asked me to provide support to the national team at the European Championships. He was part of that team and I travelled with the team and watched him win gold and the athlete of the tournament award. At the Rio Olympics 2016, I was again volunteering as a field-of-play dentist and witnessed him compete. At this Olympics though, I was now his dentist and a friend. I later found myself watching

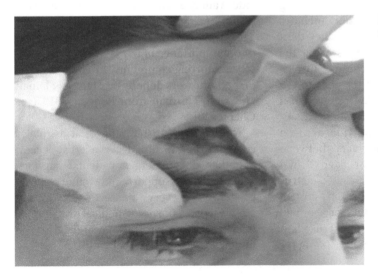

Figure 11.10 **Laceration received during competition.**

Figure 11.11 Warm-up area before competition.

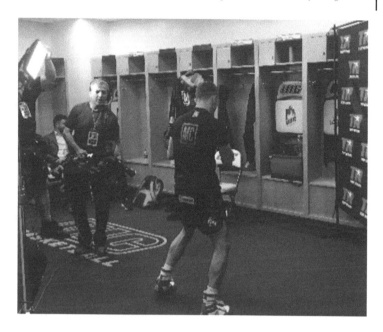

him warm up for his second profession competition in Chicago, which he was headlining (Figure 11.11). I was there as a fan. As I walked out behind him as he entered the arena, I thought of how my sports dentistry journey had brought me this fantastic experience.

So to any dentist thinking of providing sports dentistry support, choose a sport you have passion about, let the experiences and relationships that you will create be your goal, and enjoy your journey in improving the oral health of athletes.

Reference

1 Ashley, P., Cole, E., Diorio, A., Tanday, A., Needleman, I. (2014). Elite athletes and oral health: a review. *British Journal of Sports Medicine* 48(7): 561–562.

Index

Sports Dentistry: Principles and Practice, First Edition. Edited by Peter D. Fine, Chris Louca and Albert Leung.
© 2019 John Wiley & Sons Ltd. Published 2019 by John Wiley & Sons Ltd.
Companion website: www.wiley.com/go/fine/sports_dentistry

Printed in the USA/Agawam, MA
March 7, 2025

883971.003